SALIVARY GLAND CYTOLOGY

SALIVARY GLAND CYTOLOGY
A Color Atlas

Edited by

Mousa A. Al-Abbadi, MD, FIAC
Professor and Chief of Pathology
James H. Quillen VA Medical Center
East Tennessee State University
Johnson City, Tennessee, USA

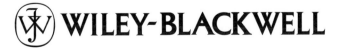

A JOHN WILEY & SONS, INC., PUBLICATION

The contents of this book do not represent the views of the Department of Veterans Affairs or the United States Government.

This work was supported by resources of the James H. Quillen VA Medical Center, Mountain Home, Tennessee, USA.

For general information on our other products and services or for technical support, please contact our Customer Care Department within the United States at (800) 762-2974, outside the United States at (317) 572-3993 or fax (317) 572-4002.

Wiley also publishes its books in a variety of electronic formats. Some content that appears in print may not be available in electronic formats. For more information about Wiley products, visit our web site at www.wiley.com.

Library of Congress Cataloging-in-Publication Data:

Salivary gland cytology : a color atlas / [edited by] Mousa A. Al-Abbadi.
         p. ; cm.
     Includes bibliographical references.
     ISBN 978-0-470-50092-7 (cloth)
     1. Salivary glands — Tumors — Cytopathology — Atlases. I. Al-Abbadi, Mousa A. [DNLM:
     1. Salivary Gland Neoplasms — pathology — Atlases. 2. Cytodiagnosis — Atlases.
     3. Salivary Gland Neoplasms — diagnosis — Atlases. 4. Salivary Glands — cytology —
     Atlases. WI 17]
     RC280.S3S25 2011
     616.99′431—dc22   2010028405

Printed in Singapore

10 9 8 7 6 5 4 3 2 1

CONTENTS

PREFACE

Real victories are those that protect human life, not those that result from its destruction or emerge from its ashes.

King Hussein

This book is dedicated to all humans suffering from the calamities of cancer. I would like specifically to devote this effort to the late King Hussein of the Hashemite Kingdom of Jordan, who succumbed to cancer. God bless his soul.

In my early professional years, I was always intrigued and fascinated by salivary gland cytology; it often appeared simple and straightforward, yet at times was very challenging. It is hoped that this first edition will help clarify, simplify, and streamline the diagnostic thought process when facing an aspirate from a salivary gland lesion. I had the good fortune to work in an institution with a very busy otolaryngology oncology service, and hence, fine needle aspiration of such lesions was very common. The wealth of the material that we studied was rich and with a broad spectrum of flavors.

All pathologists know that a very diverse group of diseases can originate from the salivary gland and that tumors from such a small organ are numerous. A great deal of overlap is evident using routine histology and even more with cytology, which led to diagnostic challenges for both the surgical pathologist and the cytopathologist alike. That is why I became interested in the subject and started the preparations to contribute with an atlas describing these lesions. The hope is to provide additional information to what has already been published about the topic. Fortunately for all of us practicing diagnosticians, only a handful of salivary gland tumors comprise the majority of neoplasms that we face. Although some pathologists are hesitant to accept fine needle aspiration biopsy as an initial diagnostic tool, we strongly believe that proper sampling and proper technique combined with the utilization of adequate clinical data provide enough ammunition to establish either a categorical or a specific diagnosis. It is hoped that this atlas, in its first edition, will help readers in their diagnostic journey of salivary gland cytology.

The readers will cruise through this atlas easily finding answers to many questions about salivary gland lesions cytology. After a brief introduction, the key cytologic diagnostic features are demonstrated followed by a differential diagnosis and clues to make a definite interpretation. The summary of these two critical issues is shown in a simple table format. A brief description of the histologic correlate with key illustrations follows. I believe that the aforementioned strategy helps resolve many questions for the clinical practitioner.

It is hoped that this book will be a positive addition and will complement many other valuable contributions on the subject by many colleagues.

I am deeply indebted to all my previous teachers and mentors who, over the years, gave me encouragement and support leading to this work. I would also like to thank all our contributors for their efforts to help make this atlas a reality. Without their efforts this would not be possible. The last chapter was not initially planned since it describes rare entities that are difficult to find. However, it was accomplished with valuable illustrations shared by our contributors.

Finally, I would like to thank all members of my family for all the support they have given me over the years.

Mousa A. Al-Abbadi

CONTRIBUTORS

MOUSA A. AL-ABBADI, MD, FIAC
Professor & Chief of Pathology
James H. Quillen VA Medical Center
East Tennessee State University
Johnson City, Tennessee 37684, USA

OZLEM E. TULUNAY-UGUR, MD
Assistant Professor & Director of Laryngology
University of Arkansas for Medical Sciences
Little Rock, Arkansas 72205, USA

IMAD ZAK, MD
Associate Professor of Radiology
Wayne State University School of Medicine
Detroit, Michigan 48201, USA

WAEL N. ZAKARIA, MD
Professor of Medicine and Infectious Diseases
James. H. Quillen VA Medical Center
East Tennessee State University
Johnson City, Tennessee 37684, USA

ISAM A. ELTOUM, MD, MBA, FIAC
Professor and Section Head of Cytopathology
University of Alabama
Birmingham, Alabama 35249, USA

JINING FENG, MD, PhD
Associate Professor of Pathology
Wayne State University
Detroit, Michigan 48201, USA

RUBA A. HALLOUSH, MD
King Hussein Cancer Center
Amman – Jordan

HUSAIN A. SALEH, MD, FIAC, MBA
Professor & Chief of Pathology
Sinai – Grace Hospital
Wayne State University
Detroit, Michigan 48235, USA

EYAS M. HATTAB, MD
Associate Professor & Director of Immunohistochemistry
Indiana University School of Medicine
Indianapolis, Indiana 46202, USA

HARVEY M. CRAMER, MD
Associate Professor & Director of Cytopathology
Indiana University School of Medicine
Indianapolis, Indiana 46202, USA

JERZY KLIJANIENKO, MD, PhD
Institut Curie
Paris – France

JAY K. WASMAN, MD
Assistant Professor of Pathology
University Hospitals Case Medical Center
Cleveland, Ohio 44106, USA

FADI W. ABDUL-KARIM, MD
Professor and Director of Anatomic Pathology
University Hospitals Case Medical Center
Cleveland, Ohio 44106, USA

PAMELA PAPAS, MD
University of Illinois Medical Center
Chicago, Illinois 60612, USA

MOMIN T. SIDDIQUI, MD, FIAC
Associate Professor & Director of Cytopathology
Emory University School of Medicine
Atlanta, Georgia 30322, USA

MOHAMMAD ABUEL-HAIJA, MD
Assistant Professor of Pathology
Indiana University School of Medicine
Indianapolis, Indiana 46202, USA

MAGDALENA CZADER, MD, PhD
Associate Professor & Director of Flow Cytometry Laboratory
Indiana University School of Medicine
Indianapolis, Indiana 46202, USA

CHAPTER 1

INTRODUCTION TO SALIVARY GLAND LESIONS CYTOLOGY

MOUSA A. AL-ABBADI, MD, FIAC

1.1 INTRODUCTION

The salivary glands are part of the exocrine secretory apparatus that are traditionally considered part of the upper gastrointestinal tract. They are a very small organ with an average total weight of 50 g in adults compared with other systems. They are composed of two major groups: the major and minor salivary glands. The major glands are composed of three paired relatively larger glands: the parotid, submandibular, and sublingual. The minor group is numerous and widely distributed in the upper aerodigestive tract (Figure 1.1).

1.2 BASIC HISTOLOGY AND PHYSIOLOGY

Salivary glands secrete digestive enzymes from their main functional unit "the acinus." The major histological components of salivary glands are as follows (Figure 1.2 illustrates these components and their cytological correlates):

1. Acinus: The main functional unit that is composed of wedge-shaped cells, each with abundant cytoplasm pushing a small round-to-oval nucleus to its periphery. They can be serous where they mainly secrete amylase, and their cytoplasm appears basophilic and densely granular with zymogen granules. These granules are periodic acid Schiff

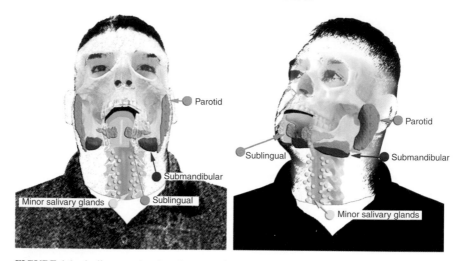

FIGURE 1.1. A diagram showing the general anatomy of salivary glands. The major salivary glands are composed of three paired, relatively larger glands: the parotid, submandibular, and sublingual. The minor salivary gland groups are numerous and widely distributed in and around the upper aerodigestive tract and are predominantly in the submucosal areas.

positive and diastase resistant. The mucinous acini secrete sialomucin, and their cytoplasm appears clear with vacuoles. The parotid gland is almost purely serous, whereas both the submandibular and the sublingual are mixed. The submandibular is more serous, and the sublingual is more mucinous.

2. Ducts: They start as small, intercalated ductules between acinar cells that are lined by single, small cuboidal cells with relatively large, centrally located nuclei. These are difficult to see on histological sections. These ductules will then join and form larger, striated ducts lined by taller columnar cells with much more abundant and eosinophilic cytoplasm rich in mitochondria. These in turn will join larger interlobar excretory ducts lined by pseudo-stratified columnar epithelium with similar features.

3. Myoepithelial cells: These stellate-shaped cells are contractile and are located outside the basement membrane of the acinar cells. They contain smooth muscle actin, myosin, and intermediate filaments such as keratin. They are difficult to see histologically.

1.3   DISEASES THAT AFFECT SALIVARY GLANDS

Many diseases can affect salivary glands. The common entities range from inflammatory/infectious non-neoplastic lesions, benign neoplasms, and

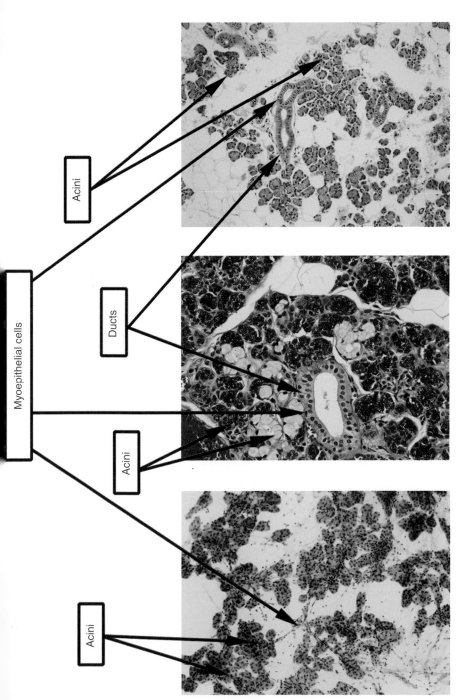

FIGURE 1.2. The three images were combined to show the three major cellular components of salivary glands. The left image is from an aspirate smear (Papanicolaou stain, 200×); the middle image is the corresponding histological section (hematoxylin and eosin, 400×); and the right image is from a cell block (hematoxylin and eosin, 200×).

TABLE 1.1. Questions to be answered when evaluating aspirates from salivary gland masses

1. Is the lesion a salivary gland lesion?
2. Is the lesion neoplastic?
3. If neoplastic, is it benign or malignant?
4. If malignant, is it high grade or low grade?
5. Can the diagnosis be specific?

malignant tumors. With an active otolaryngology service, pathologists are frequently asked to perform or interpret fine needle aspirates from salivary gland masses. Most mass lesions suspected to develop from salivary glands pose diagnostic challenges and are aspirated to determine the underlying disease process. Masses of the parotid gland are the most frequent. In these circumstances, the major questions that face pathologists are summarized in Table 1.1. Chapter 2 was written by an oncologic otolaryngology surgeon (Dr. Tulunay-Ugur) and clearly illustrates the preoperative approach of these tumors and lesions and what the surgeon would like to see in the fine needle aspiration report.

1.4 EPIDEMIOLOGY OF SALIVARY GLAND TUMORS

Despite its small size, tumors of the salivary glands are numerous and they characteristically exhibit a relatively significant degree of overlap on both morphologic and cytologic grounds. The most recent World Health Organization (WHO) list of primary tumors included 10 benign epithelial tumors, 24 malignant epithelial tumors, 1 soft tissue benign tumor (hemangioma), and lymphomas (Table 1.2). Secondary and metastatic tumors can occur, but they are less frequent and most are secondary to other head and neck neoplasms. Benign tumors are much more common than malignant ones, and the parotid gland is the most frequently involved. In addition, it is well known that the relative frequency of malignancy is inversely proportional to gland size. Therefore, malignant tumors approximately comprise 25% of parotid gland tumors, 45% of submandibular gland tumors, 80% of sublingual tumors, and 50% of minor salivary gland tumors. Therefore, extra attention has to be paid to the salient features of malignancy on cytological grounds when dealing with sublingual and minor salivary gland masses. Most tumors that occur in the floor of the mouth, the tongue, and the retro molar areas are essentially malignant. There are well-known geographic variations and gender disparities. However, these will be tackled in the following chapters. In the United States, malignancies of salivary glands comprise approximately 6% of all head and neck cancers and less than 1% of all malignancies.

TABLE 1.2. Salivary gland tumors[a]

Benign epithelial tumors:

Pleomorphic adenoma

Warthin's tumor

Myoepithelioma

Basal cell adenoma

Sebaceous adenoma

Lymphadenoma (Sebaceous and nonsebaceous)

Canalicular adenoma

Oncocytoma

Cystadenoma

Ductal papilloma (intraductal papilloma, inverted ductal papilloma, sialadenoma papilleferum)

Malignant epithelial tumors:

Mucoepidermoid carcinoma

Acinic cell carcinoma

Adenoid cystic carcinoma

Carcinoma ex pleomorphic adenoma

Polymorphous low-grade adenocarcinoma

Epithelial-myoepithelial carcinoma

Basal cell adenocarcinoma

Salivary duct carcinoma

Oncocytic carcinoma

Myoepithelial carcinoma

Clear cell carcinoma, not otherwise specified

Metastasizing pleomorphic adenoma

Small cell carcinoma

Squamous cell carcinoma

Lymphoepithelial carcinoma

Sialoblastoma

Large cell carcinoma

Cystadenocarcinoma

Low-grade cystadenocarcinoma

Mucinous adenocarcinoma

Sebaceous carcinoma

Sebaceous lymphadenocarcinoma

Carcinosarcoma

Adenocarcinoma, not otherwise specified

Soft tissue tumors: _hemangioma_

Hematolymphoid tumors: _Hodgkin's lymphoma, diffuse large cell lymphoma, extranodal marginal zone lymphoma_

Metastatic tumors

[a]Adapted from the most recent WHO classification. Lyon: IARC Press; 2005.

Overall, the most common tumor type is pleomorphic adenoma followed by Warthin's tumor. Mucoepidermoid carcinoma is the most frequent carcinoma followed by acinic cell carcinoma and adenoid cystic carcinoma. In general, tumors can occur at any age with a wide age variation; detailed descriptions of each entity will be demonstrated in the following chapters. It is important to mention that mucoepidermoid and acinic cell carcinoma are two malignancies that not uncommonly may occur in children. Figure 1.3 demonstrates major salivary gland tumors and their similarity of different cell components.

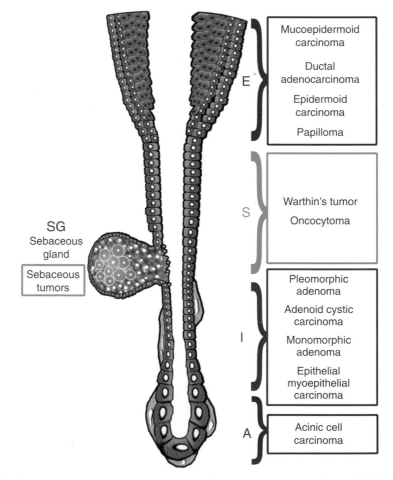

FIGURE 1.3. An illustration that shows some of the common tumors and potential similarity and proposed cell of origin. (Modified with permission from Histology for Pathologists, 2nd ed., Edited by Stephen S. Sternberg, Lippincott Williams & Wilkins, page 423.)

1.5   INDICATIONS FOR SALIVARY GLAND FINE NEEDLE ASPIRATION AND PRACTICAL CONSIDERATIONS

There is still some resistance against the concept of pretreatment fine needle aspiration (FNA) of unexplained salivary gland masses. On the one hand, the opponents of FNA argue that significant diagnostic overlap occurs among different salivary gland lesions and, ultimately, that surgical removal will be needed. On the other hand, the proponents believe that specific accurate FNA diagnosis can be reached in most cases and that surgery can be avoided in many circumstances. Scenarios where surgery can be avoided include inflammatory diseases, lymphomas, metastases, or benign neoplasms in otherwise elderly patients with multiple comorbidities. In addition, it is safe to say that even if there is no specific diagnosis, the preliminary cytological impression in most cases help guide the surgeon to determine what type of salivary gland surgery the patient will have (radical or simple excision).

Complications from salivary gland FNA are rare, and when they occur, they are not serious. Bleeding, infection, and pain from facial nerve trauma are among the most frequent. FNA-induced infarction has been reported and most commonly affects Warthin's tumor and oncocytic neoplasms. Tumor seeding is an extremely rare occurrence. No salivary gland FNA adequacy criteria have been established yet.

1.6   ACCURACY OF SALIVARY GLAND FINE NEEDLE ASPIRATION

The accuracy of FNA of salivary gland lesions is variable and depends on multiple variable factors. According to older data, the rate of correctly establishing a malignant or benign neoplasm can be achieved in more than 80% of the cases, whereas reaching a specific diagnosis ranges between 60% and 75% of the cases. However, in more recent data, the accuracy is higher where both sensitivity and sensitivity approaches more than 90%. The accuracy depends on multiple factors that include aspirator experience, availability of clinical and radiological data about the lesion, and using different types of stains of the aspirated smears. Reaching a specific diagnosis may not be possible in all cases; however, a major, categorical, nonspecific diagnosis would be extremely helpful for the treating clinicians. A diagnosis of "negative for neoplasm," "benign neoplasm," "low-grade carcinoma," or "high-grade malignancy/carcinoma" are extremely informative to surgeons. Although the accuracy of fine needle aspiration is variable and in some reports was not high enough to be acceptable, we believe that it is the best initial diagnostic approach. False-negative diagnosis can occur and results from sampling issues or interpretation. False-positive diagnosis also can occur but less frequently than false-negatives and mostly from overcalling atypia. The

TABLE 1.3. Recommendations that increase accuracy of salivary gland aspiration

1. The clinical and radiological data should be known before the procedure
2. Multiple passes should be performed in different directions (Figure 1.4)
3. Multiple stains should be used (Diff-Quik, Papanicolaou, and hematoxylin and eosin)
4. Conventional smears are preferred
5. Reaspiration of cystic lesions should be performed before its collapse (Figure 1.5)
6. Mild atypia can be seen in pleomorphic adenoma (the most common tumor of salivary glands)
7. Ancillary studies should be performed when needed at the time of aspiration (such as culture and flow cytometry)

value of a frozen section for salivary gland lesions is controversial, and in general, it is well accepted that a preoperative FNA is superior. We strongly believe that the sensitivity and specificity may be enhanced if certain precautions and steps are followed. These recommendations are as follows (Table 1.3):

1. It is advisable to have the radiological images conducted before the aspiration. The radiological information are very helpful for the aspirator; they confirm the exact location of the lesion and determine whether the lesion is in the salivary gland and shows the relation of the lesion with the surrounding structures. Chapter 3 includes more details. Furthermore, the availability of clinical data especially when the pathologists themselves perform the procedure and communicate with the patient adds an important dimension.
2. In most circumstances, one pass may not be adequate. Therefore, multiple passes in different directions are highly recommended to help sample as much as possible from the lesion. From our experience, two to four passes is usually adequate (Figure 1.4).
3. Utilization of multiple different stains is extremely critical. As many salivary gland tumors contain stroma, the presence of air-dried type smears such as Diff-Quik stain is very important. In our practice, we use Diff-Quik stain on the initial air-dried smears, Papanicolaou stain for the rest of smears, and always try to prepare the cell block. The final product that will be evaluated will include smears stained with Diff-Quik stain, Papanicolaou stain, and hematoxylin and eosin stain. Combining all these stains into a single case is valuable in interpreting salivary gland lesions.
4. Despite the shortage of data regarding using liquid-based smears in salivary gland aspiration, we strongly believe that direct conventional smears are preferred and superior.

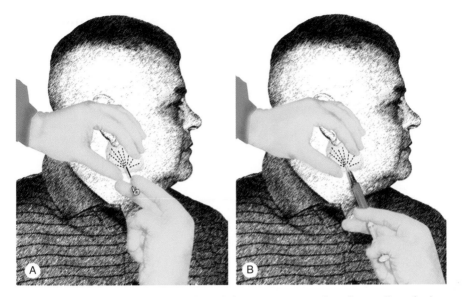

FIGURE 1.4. Diagram demonstrates the techniques we use to perform fine needle aspiration. (**a**) We prefer to start with aspiration using a needle without syringe or suction (also known as the French technique or Zajdela technique). The advantage of this technique is providing a nice, thin smear with less crush artifacts enabling the interpreter of optimum cytological morphology to proceed with appropriate triage. (**b**) The following passes can be used by employing a syringe with suction using negative pressure to increase cellularity. The aspiration can be performed with or without commercially available "guns" depending on the aspirator preference.

5. Reaspiration of cystic lesions while keeping the needle of the first pass inside the mass is a very helpful trick that helps sample the wall of the lesion and is believed to increase sensitivity (Figure 1.5).

6. Pleomorphic adenoma aspirates may show a mild degree of atypia.

7. A proper medium and tubes may be needed for ancillary studies, such as culture and immunophenotyping for lymphoid lesions.

Despite the aforementioned discussion, some lesions always pose diagnostic challenges and are problematic. The list includes basaloid tumors, lymphomas, low-grade mucoepidermoid carcinoma, acinic cell carcinoma, carcinoma ex pleomorphic adenoma, and myoepithelial cell tumors. Additionally, although not absolutely required by surgeons, establishing a specific diagnosis when dealing with high-grade carcinoma smears is sometimes impossible. These issues will be discussed in details in the following chapters.

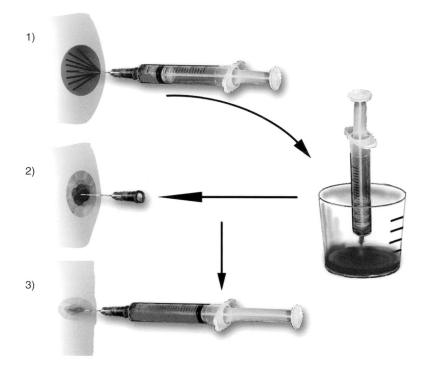

FIGURE 1.5. A diagram that shows the steps that are used when aspirating a cystic mass. Reaspiration of cystic lesions while keeping the needle of the first pass inside the mass is a very helpful trick that assist in sampling the wall of the lesion and is believed to increase sensitivity.

ACKNOWLEDGMENTS

The author would like to thank Mr. Christopher Arnold from the Medical Media section at the James H. Quillen Veteran Administration Medical Center who provided help in creating the illustrations and drawings in this chapter.

RECOMMENDED READINGS

Al-Abbadi MA. Pitfalls in Salivary gland fine-needle aspiration cytology Letter to the editor. Arch Pathol Lab Med, 2006;130:1428.

Eneroth CM, Frazen S, Zajicek J. Cytologic diagnosis of aspirate from 1000 salivary-gland tumours. Acta Otolaryngol 1966;suppl 224:168–172.

Frable MA, Frable WJ. Fine-needle aspiration biopsy of salivary glands. Laryngo-scope 1991;101:245–249.

Hughes JH, Volk EE, Wilbur DC. Pitfalls in salivary gland fine-needle aspiration cytology: lessons from the College of American Pathologists Interlaboratory

Comparison Program in Nongynecologic Cytology. Arch Pathol Lab Med 2005;129:26–31.

Layfield LJ. Fine-needle aspiration in the diagnosis of head and neck lesions: a review and discussion of problems in differential diagnosis. Diagn Cytopathol 2007;35:798–805.

Layfield LJ, Glasgow BJ. Diagnosis of salivary gland tumors by fine-needle aspiration cytology: a review of clinical utility and pitfalls. Diagn Cytopathol 1991;7:267–272.

Heller KS, Dubner S, Chess Q, Attie JN. Value of fine needle aspiration biopsy of salivary gland masses in clinical decision-making. Am J Surg 1992;164:667–670.

Rajwanshi A, Gupta K, Gupta N, Shukla R, Srinivasan R, Nijhawan R, Vasishta R. Fine-needle aspiration cytology of salivary glands: diagnsotic pitfalls re-visited. Diagn Cytopathol 2006;34:580–584.

Seethala RR, Livolsi VA, Baloch ZW. Relative accuracy of fine needle aspiration and frozen section in the diagnosis of lesions of the parotid gland. Head Neck 2005;27:217–223.

Zhang S, Bao R, Bagby J, Abre F. Fine needle aspiration of salivary glandsL 5-year experience from a single academic center. Acta Cytol 2009;53:375–382.

CHAPTER 2

SURGERY FOR SALIVARY GLAND LESIONS: A SURGEON'S PERSPECTIVE

OZLEM E. TULUNAY-UGUR, MD

2.1 SURGICAL ANATOMY

Salivary glands are composed of major and minor glands. The parotid glands (14–28 g) are the largest of the major salivary glands and are located in the preauricular region, along the posterior surface of the mandible. Although the lobes do not have distinctive separations, the parotid gland is divided by the facial nerve into a superficial lobe and a deep lobe. The superficial lobe is lateral to the nerve and the masseter muscle, whereas the deep lobe is medial to the nerve (Figure 2.1). This relationship is of outmost importance during surgery and will be discussed in detail in the following sections. The gland is located between the mastoid bone, stylomastoid process, ramus of the mandible, external acoustic meatus, and the glenoid fossa. The parotid duct—Stensen's duct—originates at the anterior border of the gland. The duct travels with the transverse facial artery, passes anterior to the masseter muscle, and then pierces the buccinator muscle to enter the oral cavity opposite to the second maxillary molar.

The second largest gland is the submandibular gland (7–8 g) located in the submandibular triangle. While the superior boundary is formed by the inferior edge of the mandible, the inferior boundaries are made up by the anterior and posterior bellies of the digastric muscle. The submandibular gland is accompanied by lymph nodes, facial artery and vein, and the lingual, hypoglossal, and mylohyoid nerves. The Wharton's duct, which is approximately 4–5 cm

Salivary Gland Cytology: A Color Atlas, Edited by Mousa A. Al-Abbadi
Copyright © 2011 Wiley-Blackwell

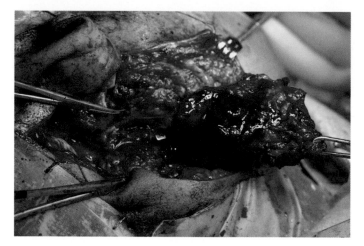

FIGURE 2.1. The mass is being lifted off of the facial nerve, which can be observed at the tip of the hemostat. The mastoid has been drilled to expose the nerve, which would otherwise be difficult to expose because of the location and size of the mass. The parotid tissue can be viewed lateral to the nerve. Partial superficial parotidectomy has been employed, and the entire nerve has not been dissected out. (Courtesy of John R. Jacobs, MD, Wayne State University)

long, empties lateral to the lingual frenulum through papilla in the floor of the mouth, on both sides of the frenulum.

The smallest major salivary gland, the sublingual gland (3 g), lies in the floor of mouth between the mucosa and the mylohyoid muscle. This gland does not have a true capsule and is medial to the mandible and genioglossus muscle. Several ducts from the superior portion of the gland either secrete directly into the floor of mouth or empty into the Bartholin's duct, which accompanies the Wharton's duct.

Approximately 600 to 1000 minor salivary glands are dispersed in the oral cavity and oropharynx. Each gland has a single duct that secretes directly into the oral cavity. They are found in the lips, gingiva, floor of the mouth, cheek, hard and soft palate, tongue, tonsils, oropharynx, larynx, and nasopharynx.

2.2   THE ROLE OF IMAGING

The most important diagnostic tool is a thorough history and physical examination. Imaging techniques play an important role in defining the extent and etiology of the disease. Imaging studies aid to define the intraglandular versus the extraglandular location of a tumor, to detect malignant features, and to assess local extension and invasion, nodal metastases, and systemic involvement. The suitable imaging technique is chosen according to the clinical picture.

Sialography relies on the injection of contrast medium into glandular ducts so that the pathway of salivary flow can be visualized by plain film radiographs. The most common indication is the presence of a calculus. Today, the use of sialographs in the clinical practice has significantly declined.

Despite being underutilized in the United States compared with Europe and Japan, ultrasound (US) is an ideal tool for initial assessment. Gritzmann (1989) reported that US was successful in defining space-occupying masses in all major salivary glands. In his study, which evaluated 302 tumors, US was able to differentiate correctly between malignant and benign lesions in 90% of the cases. It can differentiate easily between glandular and extraglandular masses and can detect the nodal status. However, it is not as useful in the delineation of deep parotid lobe masses because of the shielding effect of the mandible or of minor salivary gland lesions. Ultrasound can be used to guide fine needle aspiration biopsies from salivary gland masses.

Computed tomography (CT) is widely used in clinical practice and is generally the study of choice in the United States. CT is much more sensitive than sialography in picking up calculi as well as intrinsic and extrinsic masses. Although it cannot differentiate definitely between benign and malignant lesions, it can yield significant information that could lead the clinician toward a favored diagnosis. Malignant tumors tend to have irregular borders, infiltration into adjacent tissues, and possibly nodal spread. Low-grade malignant or benign tumors generally have regular, smooth borders and are well circumscribed. Usually, CT is accurate in differentiating deep parotid lobe tumors from other parapharyngeal masses. This distinction is important because it may change the surgical approach. Deep parotid lobe tumors displace the fat plane between the parotid and the pharyngeal constrictors medially, whereas parapharyngeal masses displace this plane laterally. The carotid artery may be displaced medially by deep lobe parotid tumors and the jugular vein by paragangliomas and schwannomas. Malignant lesions generally tend to destroy and infiltrate fascial planes.

Mandelblatt et al. (1987) reported magnetic resonance imaging (MRI) to be superior to CT in distinguishing the parotid gland from surrounding structures. In their series, MRI was also more useful in differentiating between deep lobe parotid tumors and other parapharyngeal masses. It provides useful information to differentiate between benign and malignant tumors. Malignant neoplasms have ill-defined borders and show infiltration, whereas benign lesions generally show discrete, well-defined borders. MRI is useful in evaluating the borders of a lesion and extension into surrounding tissues. The facial nerve cannot be visualized on CT but can be identified on thin section sagittal MR images.

The role of sintigraphy and positron emission tomography (PET) in the work-up of salivary gland tumors is limited. Warthin's tumor and oncocytomas are radiopositive. In salivary gland tumors, FDG-PET shows low accuracy in distinguishing benign tumors from malignancies, as benign tumors such as pleomorphic adenoma and Warthin's tumor also have a high glucose uptake. Integrated PET/CT has also been found to be poor in differentiating between benign and malignant tumors of the salivary glands. On the other hand, it can play an important role in the management of high-grade malignant tumors of salivary gland origin. Jeong et al. (2007) reported that the accuracy of PET/CT was higher than CT alone for predicting the tumor extent as well as the status of the lymph nodes in the neck. They found that with the use of PET/CT, the clinical management was modified in 43.2% of the patients, and they concluded that PET/CT provided accurate diagnostic information during the evaluation of high-grade salivary gland malignancies.

The differentiation of a benign lesion from a possible malignancy using imaging studies plays an important role not only in surgical planning but also in decision making for patients who may be poor surgical candidates. For example, an elderly patient with multiple comorbidities, who may have significant increase in mortality and morbidity during general anesthesia, may be observed in the light of radiological findings that suggest that the mass is benign. However, radiology cannot take the place of tissue diagnosis. One of the most important diagnostic tools we have in our armamentarium is fine needle aspiration biopsy, and it should be used in conjunction with imaging studies as an initial diagnostic tool. It can provide invaluable information in the management of salivary glands tumors.

2.3   FINE NEEDLE ASPIRATION

Fine needle aspiration biopsies (FNABs), which can be performed with palpation or image guidance, are becoming the standard first-line approach in the management of head and neck tumors. They are essentially safe and cost effective. Sensitivity, specificity, and diagnostic accuracy are variable and depend on multiple factors including sampling, interpretation, and whether immediate adequacy and triage evaluation was performed. In a recent study, we evaluated the factors leading to discrepant diagnosis in head and neck cancer. One of the most important factors we found leading to misdiagnosis was the lack of onsite triage at the time the FNAB procedure. A cytopathologist on site can improve sampling substantially, especially if additional material is needed for ancillary studies such as flowcytometry or immunohistochemistry. Although a routine initial FNAB is recommended by most professionals, few surgeons recommend a more selective approach. Cohen et al. (2004) recommend that FNAB be used in selected clinical scenarios. These include (1) the evaluation of poorly defined salivary gland masses, in which case if a malignancy is confirmed, then the patient can be properly counseled with regard to the extent of the surgery needed and possible risk of nerve sacrifice; (2) suspected nonsalivary pathology such as lymphoma; (3) suspected recurrent or metastatic disease; and (4) counseling and diagnosis in patients who are poor surgical

TABLE 2.1. Advantages of preoperative fine needle aspiration biopsy

1. To determine whether surgery is needed
2. To help plan for surgery
3. To counsel patients in case of malignancy
4. To avoid surgery in case of metastasis, recurrence, inflammatory diseases, and benign/low-grade lesions, lymphoms
5. To leave open the option for intraoperative fine needle aspiration and/or frozen section

candidates. They do not recommend the routine use of FNAB in well-defined masses as it usually does not alter the surgical plan or the extent of resection. Also, the management of the facial nerve is based on preoperative facial nerve function and intraoperative findings. In contrast, many studies suggest a trend toward a more liberal use of FNAB in the management of salivary gland tumors. Alphs et al. (2006) recommend to follow three principles when using FNAB in the diagnosis of parotid tumors: (1) They suggest that the primary role of a FNAB is to establish the need for definitive surgery, not to establish a specific diagnosis; (2) when decisions are being made with regard to the extent of the surgery, FNAB plays a subsidiary role to intraoperative findings; and (3) in instances where clinical impression and FNAB do not concur, intraoperative frozen section remains an important diagnostic tool. With all these in mind, it should also be remembered that well-used FNAB can prevent unnecessary surgery, or in certain instances where a malignancy was not suspected prior to the biopsy, it can result in the employment of the necessary surgical approach. One additional important advantage of having a preoperative cytopathological impression is providing the patients with objective information regarding the nature of their disorder. The information from the biopsies may also lead to further imaging studies and consultations. In a study by Heller et al. (1992), it was noted that FNAB changed the clinical approach in 35% of the patients. Examples of such changes included avoiding surgical resection for lymphomas and inflammatory masses and adapting a more conservative approach with benign tumors in the elderly and high-surgical-risk patients. Table 2.1 summarizes the advantages of having a preoperative FNA interpretation.

2.4 SALIVARY GLAND TUMORS

Salivary gland neoplasms are rare and constitute 3–4% of all head and neck tumors. The majority (70%) of the salivary gland tumors arise from the parotid glands. Although most of the minor salivary gland tumors are malignant, approximately 75% of the parotid gland tumors are benign. Pleomorphic adenoma is the most common benign tumor, followed by

Warthin's tumor. Salivary gland tumors generally have an indolent course, and are present for many years before the patient seeks medical attention with the appearance of a lump in their neck or face. The most common presenting symptom is painless swelling. Pain is generally a sign of an inflammatory process. Bilateral masses are not common but can be viewed as a result of autoimmune disease or caused by cystic degeneration in patients with HIV. A recent increase in the size of a mass that has been stable for many years or the recent onset of pain and facial nerve weakness should raise suspicion of malignancy. History of skin cancer needs to be questioned because of the risk of metastasis to the parotid.

Examination usually reveals a nontender, mobile, and well-defined mass. Similar to facial nerve weakness, fixation to the adjacent structures or the presence of cervical lymphadenopathy may be signs of a malignancy. Minor salivary gland tumors generally present as normal mucosa-covered masses in their corresponding anatomical location. Malignant tumors of the submandibular glands can present with weakness of the marginal mandibular nerve with drooping at the corner of the lip or ipsilateral weakness or numbness of the tongue as a result of the involvement of the hypoglossal and lingual nerves. Sudden painful swelling of the submandibular gland also occurs commonly because of sialolithiasis.

2.5   SURGICAL APPROACH

The management of the salivary gland neoplasms depends on the location of the tumor and the histology. In the parotid gland, surgical approaches include a partial or complete superficial parotidectomy (SP), total parotidectomy (TP), or a radical parotidectomy (RP). In partial superficial parotidectomy the tumor localized in the superficial lobe is resected with a surrounding 1–2 cm cuff of normal parotid tissue, compared with removing the entire superficial lobe in a complete SP (Figure 2.1). Similarly, in TP the facial nerve is preserved compared with an RP where the nerve is sacrificed. A partial SP results in the avoidance of unnecessary dissection of the facial nerve. For example, a tumor at the tail of the parotid gland may be excised just by dissecting the lower division of the nerve that preserves the upper division of the facial nerve. In a recent study, it has been shown that complete SP results in higher rates of transient facial nerve dysfunction and Frey's syndrome. On the other hand, simple enucleation is discouraged because of the high risk of recurrence. Larger tumors of the parotid gland may require a complete SP and deep lobe tumors are excised by a TP.

The submandibular gland is excised through a transcervical approach. The marginal mandibular branch of the facial nerve lies in the fascia superficial to the gland. This fascia is retracted superiorly so that the nerve can be preserved. The hypoglossal nerve and the lingual nerve lie underneath the gland and unless involved with tumor; these are preserved as well. In case of malignancy, the excision can be extended to involve the surrounding muscles and mandibulectomy.

The extent of resection and the approach for minor salivary gland tumors will depend on the location of the tumor. The T staging for these tumors is also performed according to the site they are localized in, e.g., oropharyngeal T staging is used.

The main controversies with regard to surgery in the treatment of salivary gland malignancies are the role of neck dissection and the indications to sacrifice the facial nerve. Most authors would agree that facial nerve sacrifice is not routinely indicated. Generally, the nerve is preserved unless there is direct extension by the tumor. If the nerve is resected, then it is grafted at the same time generally by using the greater auricular or sural nerve. Postoperative radiotherapy is not a contraindication for nerve grafting and does not impair nerve healing. It is likely that the function of the grafted segment will not return to normal volitional activity, but improved tone will aid in the rehabilitative effort.

Patients with malignant tumors who present with lymphadenopathy undergo a therapeutic neck dissection. The management is debated in patients with no clinically enlarged lymph nodes (by clinical examination and radiological imaging). Zbären et al. (2005) retrospectively analyzed the outcome of 83 patients treated for a parotid gland malignancy. Approximately half of the patients underwent an elective neck dissection (ND) and the other half was observed. Occult metastasis was detected in 20% of the patients. Locoregional recurrence was noted in 12% of the patients in the elective ND group compared with 26% of the observation group, and all neck recurrences were found in the observation-only group. However, although the disease-free survival was longer in the elective ND group, the overall survival was not significantly different among both groups. Nonetheless, they recommend an elective ND in all parotid gland malignancies. Furthermore, Medina (1998) summarized the indications for an elective neck dissection as follows: high grade tumors, T3 and T4 tumors, tumors larger than 3 cm, presence of facial nerve paralysis, patients older than 54 years old, extraglandular extension, and perilymphatic invasion. Most patients will fail because of distant metastasis rather than local failure. By most surgeons, an elective ND is employed including levels I through III for tumors larger than 4 cm, squamous cell carcinoma, adenocarcinoma, undifferentiated carcinoma, and high-grade mucoepidermoid carcinoma.

2.6   ROLE OF FROZEN SECTION (FS) ANALYSIS

The main indications for FS include the following: detecting free margins, detecting involvement of the nerve, detecting involvement of the lymph nodes, ensuring adequate resection, preventing overaggressive surgery, and occasionally, confirming or obtaining a diagnosis. The published reports on the accuracy of FS in salivary gland tumors are inconsistent. Megerian and Maniglia (1994) reported a diagnostic accuracy of 94.1% with a 2.1% false positivity and 8.8% false negativity rate. In the series by Rigaul et al., accuracy is 92% and the false positivity and negativity are 2% each. Wong (2002) reported similar results in terms of accuracy of an FS to differentiate between a benign and malignant tumor at 94.7%. The sensitivity for a malignancy was 100% and specificity 87.5%. The false positivity rate was 12.5% and false negativity was 0%. In this series, a pleomorphic adenoma case was misdiagnosed and reported as a malignancy out of 19 cases sent to confirm diagnosis. Margins were assessed by FS in 15 cases, and of these, in two cases the margins were reported incorrectly as no evidence of tumor because of sampling error. Eight cases were referred to evaluate nerve involvement, one case was reported as suspicious for malignancy (the pleomorphic adenoma case reported falsely as malignant), and nerve sacrifice was not performed because of the lack of informed consent. This report draws attention to all of the pitfalls of FS diagnosis. The role of cautious clinical interpretation cannot be over-emphasized. Good communication between the surgeon and the pathologist is of outmost importance. It can be devastating to base the clinical decision making solely on the FS report, which needs to be incorporated into the entire clinical picture.

2.7 COMPLICATIONS OF SALIVARY GLAND SURGERIES

Facial nerve paralysis is one of the most devastating complications. If accidental transaction of the nerve is recognized, it is repaired before awakening the patient. Gustatory sweating or Frey's syndrome occurs at varying degrees after parotidectomy. Most patients would be asymptomatic, although a small group of patients can be significantly affected socially. It is believed that the postganglionic parasympathetic fibers grow into the dermis and innervate the sweat glands. Therefore, the patient complains of sweating at that side of the face once they start eating. Prevention can be attempted by placing acellular dermis, fat grafting, or by using flaps. Symptomatic patients can be treated with injection of Botox into the affected area, the application of topical glycopyrrolate cream, or the use of antiperspirants. If these measures are not successful, surgery can be employed by either placing a flap underlying the skin or by performing a tympanic neurectomy. Hematoma or seroma are two of the most frequent complications and can lead to wound infection or, rarely, compression of the nerve; therefore, they need to be evacuated when recognized. Meticulous hemostasis should be performed to avoid them.

Submandibular gland surgeries can result in the injury of the marginal mandibular branch of the facial nerve, which would result in drooping of the lip.

Injury to the lingual nerve leading to numbness of the tongue or injury to the hypoglossal nerve resulting in immobility of that side of the tongue can also be observed.

Complications of surgeries for minor salivary glands would depend on the location of the tumor.

RECOMMENDED READINGS

Alphs HH, Eisele DW, Westra WH. The role of fine needle aspiration in the evaluation of parotid masses. Curr Opin Otolaryngol Head Neck Surg 2006;14 (2):62–66.

Cohen EG, Patel SG, Lin O, Boyle JO, Kraus DH, Singh B, Wong RJ, Shah JP, Shaha AR. Fine-needle aspiration biopsy of salivary gland lesions in a selected patient population. Arch Otolaryngol Head Neck Surg 2004;130(6):773–778.

Cummings CW, Flint PW, Haughey BH, et al., editors. Otolaryngology Head and Neck Surgery. 4th ed. St. Louis (MO): Mosby; 2005.

Gritzmann N. Sonography of the salivary glands. Am J Roentgenol 1989;153: 161–166.

Heller KS, Dubner S, Chess Q, Attie JN. Value of fine needle aspiration biopsy of salivary gland masses in clinical decision-making. Am J Surg 1992;164:667–670.

Jeong HS, Chung MK, Son YI, Choi JY, Kim HJ, Ko YH, Baek CH. Role of 18F-FDG PET/CT in management of high-grade salivary gland malignancies. J Nucl Med 2007;48(8):1237–1244.

Lee YY, Wong KT, King AD, Ahuja AT. Imaging of salivary gland tumors. Eur J Radiol 2008;66(3):419–436.

Mandelblatt SM, Braun IF, Davis PC, Fry SM, Jacobs LH, Hoffman JC Jr. Parotid masses: MR imaging. Radiology 1987;163(2):411–414.

Medina JE. Neck dissection in the treatment of cancer of major salivary glands. Otolaryngol Clin North Am 1998;31(5):815–822.

Megerian CA, Maniglia AJ. Parotidectomy: a ten year experience with fine needle aspiration and frozen section biopsy correlation. Ear Nose Throat J 1994;73 (6):377–380.

Myers EN, Ferris RL, editors. Salivary Gland Disorders. Berlin (Germany): Springer; 2007.

Wong DS. Frozen section during parotid surgery revisited: efficacy of its applications and changing trend of indications. Head Neck 2002;24(2):191–197.

Zbären P, Schüpbach J, Nuyens M, Stauffer E. Elective neck dissection versus observation in primary parotid carcinoma. Otolaryngol Head Neck Surg 2005;132(3):387–391.

CHAPTER 3

RADIOLOGICAL INVESTIGATION OF SALIVARY GLAND LESIONS

IMAD ZAK, MD

3.1 INTRODUCTION

Imaging plays a major role in the management of patients with head and neck tumors, which includes tumors developing in the salivary glands. Imaging can define the location, origin, and frequently the nature of the mass lesion. It also aids in the staging of head and neck cancer.

3.2 OVERVIEW OF IMAGING MODALITIES

Currently, a variety of imaging modalities are often used for evaluating the major salivary glands. The most common in our practice is contrast enhanced computerized tomography (CT) of the entire neck obtained on a multidetector CT scanner. A volume of data at 0.6-mm isometric voxels is acquired from the level of sella turcica to the level of aortopulmonary window. Axial images are then reconstructed using soft tissue and bone window algorithms at 3-mm intervals. Reformations are obtained routinely in the coronal and sagittal planes at 3-mm intervals.

CT remains the modality of choice for the initial assessment of head and neck cancer. It provides valuable information about the location, margins, size, and extent of the tumor. Additionally, CT is the best available imaging modality for detection of calcifications and stones (Figure 3.1).

The second most common modality in our practice is magnetic resonance imaging (MRI). In a few situations, MRI is the modality of choice in

Salivary Gland Cytology: A Color Atlas, Edited by Mousa A. Al-Abbadi
Copyright © 2011 Wiley-Blackwell

TABLE 3.1. Imaging modalities in common use			
Imaging modality	CT	MRI	US
Risks/ disadvantages	• Ionizing radiation	• Ferromagnetic attraction • Heat and current loops	• Safe • Operator dependent
Advantages	• Fast • Widely available	• Limited availability	• Widely available
Cost	• Intermediate cost	• Expensive	• Low cost
Indications	• Initial evaluation • Calcifications, stones • Guidance for deep biopsy	• Tissue characterization • Floor of mouth invasion • Perineural spread • Skull base invasion	• Cyst versus solid tumor • Guidance for superficial biopsy

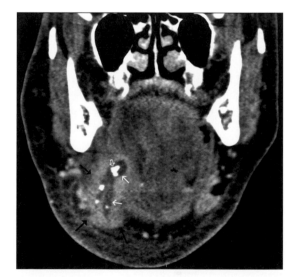

FIGURE 3.1. Sialoadenitis of right submandibular gland. Coronal CT scan shows enlarged right submandibular gland (long black arrows) with edema of the adjacent tissue planes. There are dilated ducts (short white arrows) with multiple stones (open arrow).

evaluating salivary gland lesions. We may begin our initial evaluation with MRI if there is a high clinical suspicion of malignancy based on a hard, rapidly growing mass in an adult patient and especially when cranial nerve palsy is present. We tailor the MRI study according to the region of interest. Typically, we acquire axial and coronal T1 weighted images (T1WI) at 4-mm intervals with a 10% gap, coronal T2 weighted images (T2WI) with fat suppression at 4-mm intervals with a 10% gap, and axial T2WI at 4-mm intervals with a 10% gap; finally, we inject intravenous gadolinium-based contrast material and acquire fat-suppressed coronal and axial T1WI with a 10% gap. Diffusion weighted imaging (DWI) is advantageous in predicting malignant versus reactive lymphadenopathy in the neck.

Because of its exquisite tissue contrast and multiplanar capabilities, MRI is the study of choice in evaluating the presence of perineural spread of tumor, violation of the adjacent tissue planes, and invasion of the skull base (Figure 3.2). Unenhanced T1WIs show a relatively dark tumor signal against a bright, fatty background especially in the parotid gland. Fat suppression techniques become necessary when contrast material (gadolinium) is used. T2WIs are useful in evaluating cysts and in detecting the cystic components associated with some solid tumors. Cysts appear well defined with a bright

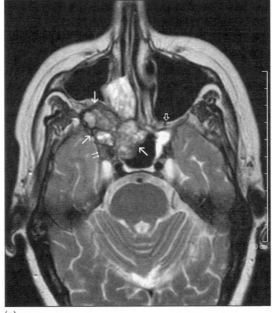

(a)

FIGURE 3.2. (*Continued*)

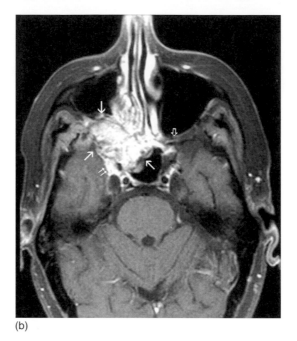

(b)

FIGURE 3.2. Adenocystic carcinoma of right ehmoid and shenoid sinuses. (a) Axial T2WI shows heterogeneous tumor with relative dark T2 signal (long white arrows). The tumor invades the right pterygopalatine fossa with intracranial extension along the trigeminal nerve. The right cavernous sinus is filled with tumor (double short white arrows). Notice normal contralateral pterygopalatine fossa (open arrow). (b) Postcontrast T1WI shows heterogeneous enhancement of the mass and better visualization of intracranial invasion.

signal on T2WI and a dark signal on T1WI (Figure 3.3). Benign lesions tend to be well defined with a relatively bright signal on T2WI (Figure 3.4), which is in contradistinction to malignant tumors that tend to have a relatively dark signal on T2WI (Figure 3.5).

Ultrasound (US) is used in some practices as the initial modality in evaluating major salivary glands, reserving other modalities for subsequent assessment. US is useful in differentiating the solid versus cystic nature of accessible head and neck lesions. It might also provide guidance for needle aspiration biopsy. In our institutions, most deep neck and parotid masses are sampled under CT guidance.

Lymphatic spread is not a common path for metastasis in salivary gland malignancy. Positron emission tomography (PET) with or without CT is implemented commonly in our institution for staging and initial evaluation of distant metastatic disease (Figure 3.6). Nuclear medicine techniques have limited use in localized salivary gland disease. Sodium pertechnitate is concentrated and subsequently secreted by the major salivary glands.

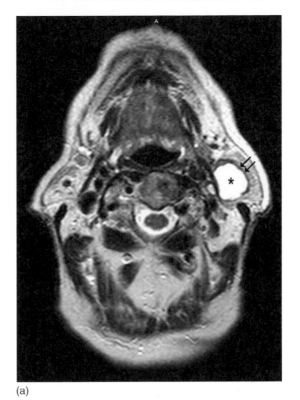

(a)

FIGURE 3.3. (*Continued*)

A Tc-99m sodium pertechnitate scan can be useful in confirming the presence or absence of normal salivary glandular tissue.

Sialography is rarely used to assess major salivary gland pathology. Painful glands should be imaged first with unenhanced CT to evaluate for the presence of ductal stones or sialolithiasis. Typically, sialography is reserved for noncalculous recurrent sialadenitis. The procedure is invasive and implies probing, cannulating, and injecting contrast material directly into Stensen or Wharton ducts. Conventional sialography is particularly useful in demonstrating sialectasis. MRI has been advocated as a potential alternative to sialography. The ability to demonstrate fluid in dilated ducts without the need for injecting contrast material is a potential major advantage of MRI (Figure 3.7).

3.3 ANATOMICAL AND PATHOLOGICAL CONSIDERATIONS

The salivary glands are divided into major and minor groups. The three pairs of major salivary glands are parotid, submandibular, and sublingual.

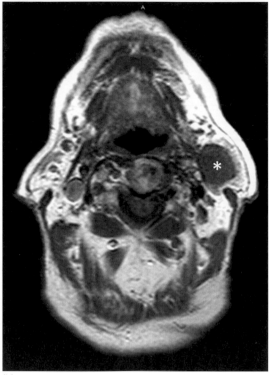

(b)

FIGURE 3.3. (*Continued*)

Innumerable minor salivary glands are found in the mucosa throughout the aero-digestive tract, including the paranasal sinuses and parapharyngeal space. Sialography is useful in evaluating ductal disease in the parotid and submandibular salivary glands by injecting iodinated contrast material into Stensen and Wharton ducts, respectively. Sialography has no role in evaluating the sublingual salivary glands. The sublingual salivary glands open directly into the floor of mouth through numerous ductules.

Warthin's tumor, intraglandular lymph nodes, and lymphoepithelial lesions of AIDS are exclusive to the parotid gland because the parotid gland encapsulates late in the second trimester after the development of the lymphatic system, whereas the submandibular and sublingual salivary glands attain capsules earlier and prior to the development of the reticuloendothelial system.

An inverse relationship exists between the size of the gland and the rate of malignancy. Benign tumors tend to occur in larger salivary glands, whereas malignant tumors are encountered more frequently in minor salivary glands.

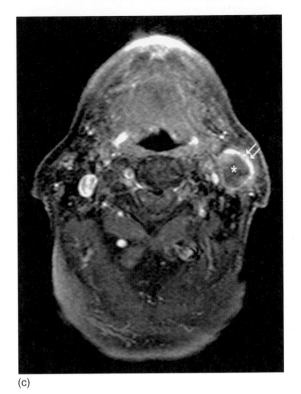

(c)

FIGURE 3.3. First branchial cleft cyst of parotid gland. (**a**) Axial T2WI shows a cystic lesion in the left parotid gland with bright contents (asterisk) and irregular dark capsule (black arrows). (**b**) Axial T1WI shows dark signal of the cyst (asterisk) in the background of bright fat containing normal parotid tissue. (**c**) Axial post contrast T1WI shows enhancement of the cyst wall (black arrows) while the cyst contents (asterisk) do not enhance.

The intraparotid facial nerve segment runs in a plane between the superficial and deep lobes. It is not advisable to perform biopsy on parapharyngeal or deep parotid lesions through a direct lateral approach. In our institution, we use a trans-buccal approach to minimize the damage to facial nerve and carotid sheath (Figure 3.8).

3.3.1 Image Interpretation and Differential Diagnosis

The current conventional wisdom is as follows: "All solitary salivary gland masses are neoplastic until proven otherwise and require fine needle aspiration biopsy." Whenever malignancy is discovered, MRI should be performed to assess invasion of adjacent tissue planes and perineural spread of tumor (Figure 3.9). Occasionally, a CT may show remodeling or

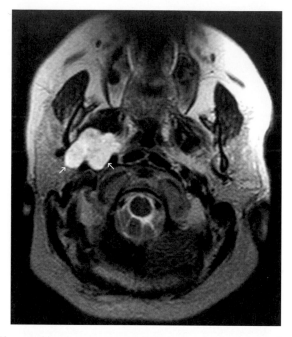

FIGURE 3.4. Pleomorphic adenoma. Axial T2WI shows a bright, lobulated, and well-defined tumor in the deep lobe of the parotid gland (white arrows).

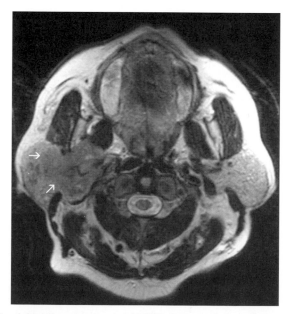

FIGURE 3.5. Basaloid cell carcinoma. Axial T2WI shows a relatively dark and poorly defined tumor in the parotid gland (white arrows).

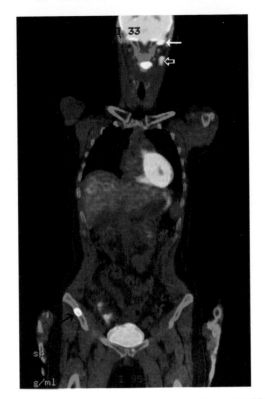

FIGURE 3.6. Adenocystic carcinoma of left parotid gland. Coronal PET-CT shows a fused PET image on a coronal reformatted CT image. High activity is observed in the left parotid gland (white arrow), metastatic left neck lymph node (open arrow), and a distant metastasis in the right iliac bone (black arrow).

destruction of skull bones (Figure 3.10). MRI is the investigation of choice for minor salivary gland disease because of a greater propensity to develop malignant tumors in the smaller glands.

A nodal or non-nodal extraglandular lesion, such as a schwannoma, masseteric hypertrophy, a primary or secondary lesion of the mandible, or a subcutaneous lesion, may be mistaken for a glandular process, even by experienced otorhinolaryngologists. Recently, we published a case of hepatocellular carcinoma metastasis to the mandible masquerading clinically as a parotid tumor (Figure 3.11).

A cyst in a major salivary gland can be mistaken clinically for a tumor. However, imaging can distinguish cysts from solid tumors easily using either ultrasound US or MRI. On US, a cyst is usually dark, well defined, round, or ovoid, and it shows a brighter posterior wall due to a phenomenon called through transmission. On the contrary, a solid tumor tends to be echogenic and lacks through transmission. Cysts are typically isointense to

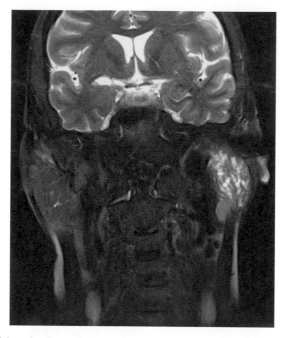

FIGURE 3.7. Sialectasis. Cononal T2WI shows branching bright tubular structures in the left parotid gland representing dilated parotid ductal system.

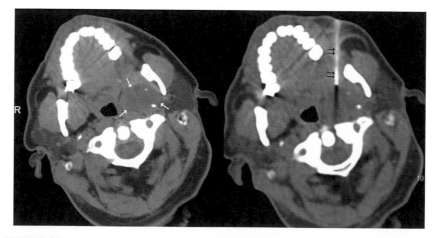

FIGURE 3.8. Acinic cell carcinoma of left parotid gland. Axial CT scan study during biopsy of a deep left parotid mass (white arrows). Notice the needle was introduced through the trans-buccal approach (black arrows).

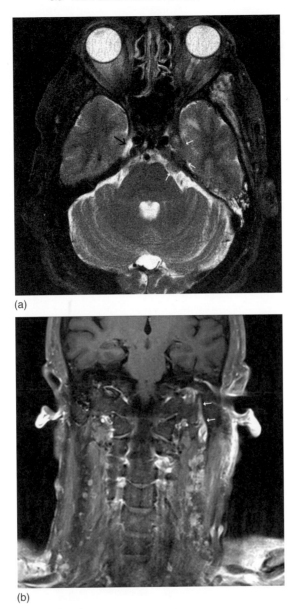

(a)

(b)

FIGURE 3.9. (a) Axial T2WI shows a tumor of dark signal in the left cavernous sinus and Mekel cave (white arrows) representing a perineural spread of adenocystic carcinoma originated in the upper lip. Notice the normal right Mickel cave (black arrow). (b) Coronal postcontrast T1WI shows enhancing tumor along the mastoid segment of the left facial nerve representing perineural spread of adenoid cystic carcinoma of the left parotid gland (white arrows)

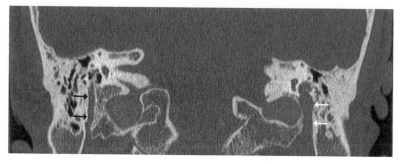

FIGURE 3.10. Cononal CT reformatted image shows enlarged vertical segment of left facial nerve canal (white arrows) caused by perineural tumor spread of the left parotid adenoid cystic carcinoma. Notice normal right facial nerve canal (black arrows).

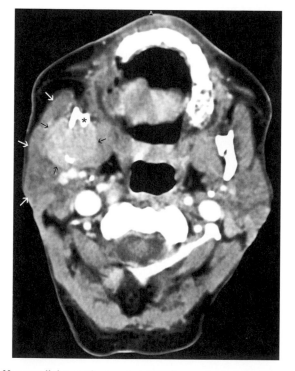

FIGURE 3.11. Hepatocellular carcinoma. Axial CT image shows enhancing metastatic tumor (black arrows) in the right masticator space deep to the parotid gland (white arrows). The tumor arises from and destroys the right mandibular ramus (asterisk).

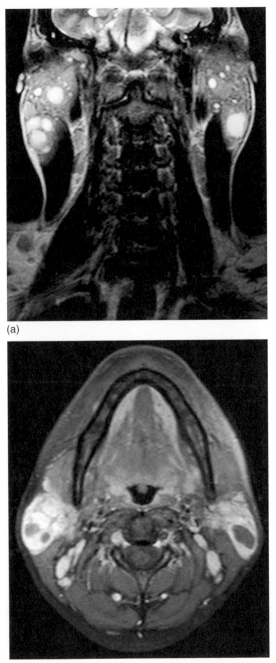

(a)

(b)

FIGURE 3.12. Lymphoepithelial lesions of AIDS. (**a**) Coronal T2WI and (**b**) Axial postcontrast T1WI show multiple bilateral cysts. Cysts appear bright on T2 and dark on T1, similar to the CSF.

cerebrospinal fluid (CSF) on all MRI sequences. Additionally, solid tumors typically enhance to some degree on both CT and MRI, whereas the cystic contents do not (Figures 3.3 and 3.12).

The superficial lobe of the parotid gland and the submandibular gland are amenable to US examination. US may not assess the deep lobe of the parotid gland and the sublingual gland adequately. For deep head and neck lesions, we prefer CT or MRI.

Diffuse multiglandular parenchymal disease can be caused by a myriad of pathology, such as viral sialadenitis, Sjögren syndrome, sarcoidosis, and benign lymphoepithelial cysts in patients with AIDS (Figure 3.12). There is an increased risk of mucosa-associated lymphoid tissue (MALT) lymphoma of the salivary glands in Sjögren syndrome. Thus, any dominant mass lesion should undergo biopsy.

Multiple masses within the parotid gland usually represent intraparotid lymph nodes. Bilateral Warthin's tumor (cystadenoma lymphomatosum) occurs in up to 20% of patients (Figure 3.13). Lymphoepithelial lesions in

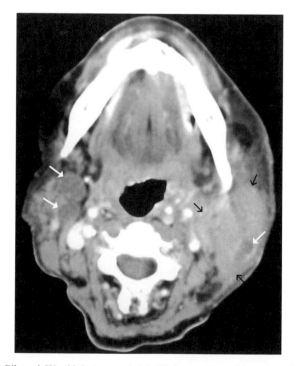

FIGURE 3.13. Bilateral Warthin's tumor. Axial CT image shows bilateral cystic lesions (white arrows) and a large solid component in the left parotid gland (black arrows).

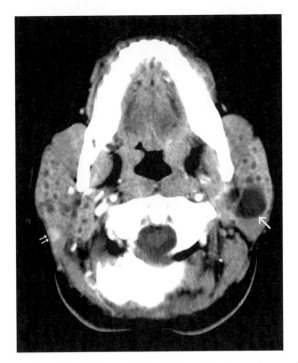

FIGURE 3.14. Lymphoepithelial lesions of AIDS. Axial CT image shows enlarged bilateral parotid glands with numerous variable-sized cysts (long white arrow) and small solid components (short double arrows). The findings are typical of lymphoepithelial lesions.

patients with AIDS might present with similar imaging characteristics (Figure 3.14). The clinical history and presence of lymphoid hyperplasia elsewhere should not pose difficulty in diagnosis. A unilateral, nonenhancing cystic mass with a high T2 signal is more likely to be a Warthin's tumor and less likely a necrotic lymph node. On the one hand, if a well-defined unilateral tumor has a high T2 signal and enhances well with contrast, then it is most likely to be a pleomorphic adenoma (Figures 3.4 and 3.15). On the other hand, if a poorly defined tumor shows a low T2 signal with or without invasion of surrounding tissue planes, then it is more likely to be a malignant tumor such as adenoid cystic carcinoma or mucoepidermoid carcinoma (Figures 3.5 and 3.16). A definitive diagnosis can only be made with tissue sampling. Pathological diagnosis by fine needle aspiration, or incisional or excisional biopsy, remains the gold standard for diagnosis of head and neck cancer and cannot be replaced by MRI.

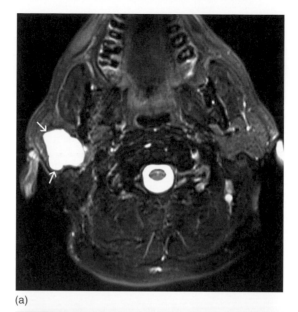

(a)

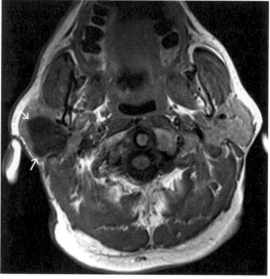

(b)

FIGURE 3.15. (*Continued*)

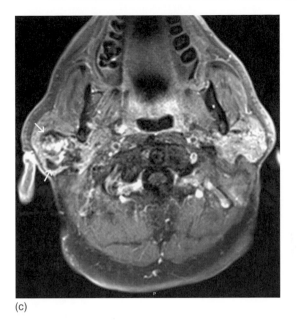

(c)

FIGURE 3.15. Pleomorphic adenoma. (**a**) Axial T2WI shows a bright and well-defined tumor (white arrows) in the right parotid gland. (**b**) Axial T1WI shows a well-defined, relatively dark tumor (white arrows) in the bright background of fatty parotid tissue. (**c**) Axial T1WI post contrast shows heterogeneous enhancement.

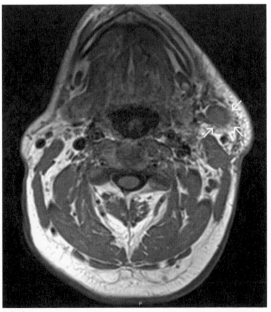

(a)

FIGURE 3.16. (*Continued*)

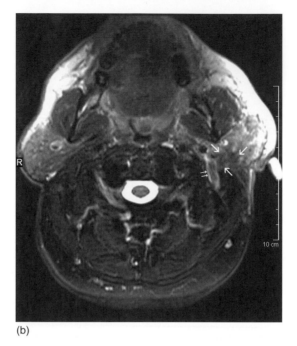

(b)

FIGURE 3.16. Adenoid cystic carcinoma. (**a**) Axial T1WI shows a poorly defined tumor with irregular posterior borders (white arrows). (**b**) Axial T2WI at the skull base shows the poorly defined tumor of low T2 signal (long white arrows) with invasion along the left facial nerve (double short white arrows).

TABLE 3.2. Appearance of salivary gland lesions on different imaging modalities

	CT	MRI	US
Cyst	• Well defined • Round • Homogeneous • No enhancement of contents	• Well defined • Round • Bright on T2WI • Dark on T1WI2 • No enhancement of contents	• Dark (anechoic) • Round compressable • Well circumscribed • Through transmission
Benign tumor	• Well defined • Dense tissue • Variable enhancement	• Well defined • Bright on T2WI • Low signal on T1WI • Intense enhancement	• Echogenic • Well circumscribed
Malignant tumor	• Poorly defined • Variable enhancement	• Irregular outline • Low signal on T2WI • Enhances with contrast	• Echogenic • Irregular outline

RECOMMENDED READINGS

Batsakis JG. Tumors of the head and neck: clinical and pathological considerations. Baltimore (MD): Williams & Wilkins; 1979.

Han L, Bhan R, Zak I, Husain M, Feng J, Vella S, Al-Abbadi M. Metastatic hepatocellular carcinoma to the mandible masquerading as a parotid gland mass: a potential pitfall in the diagnosis by fine needle aspiration biopsy. Diagn Cytopathol 2007;35(10):674–676.

Higashino H, Horii T, Ohkusa Y, Ohkuma H, Ino C, Nakazawa M, Izumi H, Kobayashi Y. Congenital absence of lacrimal puncta and of all major salivary glands: case report and literature review. Clin Pediatr 1987;26(7): 366–368.

Liyanage SH, Spencer SP, Hogarth KM, Makdissi J. Imaging of salivary glands. Imaging 2007;19:14–27.

MRI sialography.

Nishimura M, Miyajima S, Okada N. Salivary gland MALT lymphoma associated with helicobacter pylori infection in a patient with Sjoegren's syndrome. J Dermatol 2000;27(7):450–452.

Rudack C, Jörg S, Kloska S, Stoll W, Thiede O. Neither MRI, CT nor US is superior to diagnose tumors in the salivary glands: an extended case study. Head Face Med 2007;3:19.

Shah GV. MR imaging of salivary glands. Magn Reson Imaging Clin N Am 2002;10 (4):631–662.

Sucupira MS, Weinreb JW, Camargo EE, Wagner HN. Salivary gland imaging and radionuclide dacryocystography in agenesis of salivary glands. Arch Otolaryngol 1983;109(3):197–198.

Sumi M, Sakihama N, Sumi T, Morikawa M, Uetani M, Kabasawa H, Shigeno K, Hayashi K, Takahashi H, Nakamura T. Discrimination of metastatic cervical lymph nodes with diffusion-weighted MR imaging in patients with head and neck cancer. Am J Neuroradiol 2003;24(8):1627–1634.

Weissman JL, Carrau RL. Anterior facial vein and submandibular gland together: predicting the histology of submandibular masses with CT or MR imaging. Radiology 1998;208:441–446.

Yousem DM, Kraut MA, Chalian AA. Major salivary gland imaging. Radiology 2000;216(1):19–29.

CHAPTER 4

INFECTIOUS AND INFLAMMATORY DISEASES OF SALIVARY GLANDS

WAEL N. ZAKARIA, MD, ISAM A. ELTOUM, MD, MBA, FIAC and
MOUSA A. AL-ABBADI, MD, FIAC

4.1 INTRODUCTION

Most of these lesions are diagnosed clinically and would not be subject to fine needle aspiration biopsy (FNAB) sampling. However, sometimes they pose diagnostic challenges radiologically and clinically, and consequently in these occasions, FNAB will be used as an initial diagnostic tool. In these circumstances, the main goal is to exclude the presence of neoplastic processes. The list is large, and many entities currently are rare. Detailed clinical descriptions are best found in textbooks of otolaryngology and infectious diseases.

4.2 ACUTE SIALADENITIS/PAROTITIS

Acute bacterial parotitis is now considered an infrequent illness, but it is still observed in the elderly, as well as in dehydrated, malnourished, and intubated patients. It is more common in children than in adults. Typical organisms cultured from those patients include *Staphylococcus aureus*, oral cavity flora, *Eikenella corrodens*, Enterobacteriaceae, and other gram-negative bacilli. Usually, the clinical presentation of acute bacterial parotitis is sudden onset of pain and local swelling over the parotid gland. Trismus, dysphagia, high fever, and toxic appearance also are common features. Physical examination

Salivary Gland Cytology: A Color Atlas, Edited by Mousa A. Al-Abbadi
Copyright © 2011 Wiley-Blackwell

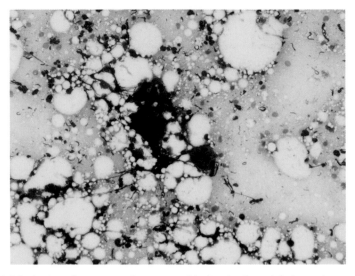

FIGURE 4.1. Aspirate from a case of acute parotitis showing few acini observed surrounded by debris and neutrophils (Diff Quik stain, 400×).

rarely yields fluctuance, but it is necessary to look for expressing pus through the Stensen duct using bimanual examination. This test might be painful, so preparing the patient will always help. In rare circumstances, the disease process may be complicated by pharyngeal obstruction, osteomyelitis, and sepsis. Obstruction from a stone in the ducts may lead to chronic sialadenitis. The diseases can present with enlargement of the gland, which can be focal or diffuse and can be either unilateral or bilateral. If FNAB is performed, usually it yields morphological features of an abscess in the form of numerous neutrophils, fibrin, crush artifacts, and sometimes evidence of necrosis (Figures 4.1 through 4.3). The fluid should be sent for culture and sensitivity. As the disease progresses, the aspirate smears will show more chronic inflammatory cells, such as lymphocytes, plasma cells, and rarely, granulation tissue formation. The diagnosis in the acute phase is straightforward, whereas the differential diagnosis in chronic and organizing phases includes lymphoepithelial lesions (lymphoepithelial sialadenitis [LES]) that may occur in HIV-positive patients (LES of AIDS [LESA]) or lymphoproliferative disorders. The former would be clear from the history, and the latter would need immunophenotypic analysis by flowcytometry on the aspirate or immunohistochemistry on cell block material.

4.3 ACUTE SIALADENITIS/PAROTITIS OF THE NEONATE

Acute parotitis of the neonate is a rare form of parotitis, which occurs usually in a premature baby with unilateral parotid swelling and inflammation. It

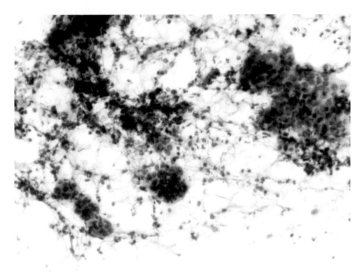

FIGURE 4.2. Multiple acini with crush artifacts surrounded by numerous neutrophils (Papanicolaou stain, 400×).

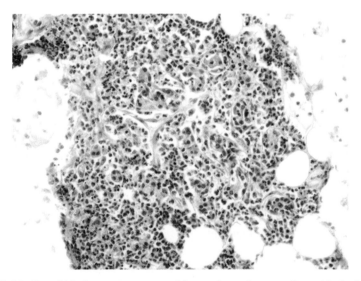

FIGURE 4.3. On cell block, numerous neutrophils are observed surrounding residual acini, some of which are completely destroyed by the acute inflammatory process. This patient was sick in the intensive care unit where the culture revealed Methicillin-resistant *S. aureus* (cell block, hematoxylin and eosin stain, 400×).

mostly occurs in male children with *S. aureus* as the most common isolate (more than 50% of the cases). Although it is extremely rare to aspirate such lesions, when performed, the aspirates contain normal salivary gland cells with increased numbers of neutrophils. Acute parotitis of the neonate is treated by systemic antibiotics, and surgery is indicated only if aggressive medical therapy fails.

4.4 CHRONIC BACTERIAL PAROTITIS

Chronic bacterial parotitis occurs in the presence of calculi, stenosis of the duct secondary to trauma, and/or in association with autoimmune processes with superimposed bacterial infection. These are rarely aspirated, but when they are, fragments of stones and chronic inflammatory cells might be observed. The differential diagnosis includes lymphoproliferative disorders in which the aspirates contain monotonous lymphoid cells, and an immuno-phenotypic analysis would be necessary to clarify the neoplastic nature of these lymphoid cells.

4.5 CHRONIC SIALADENITIS

Chronic sialadenitis is more common in the submandibular glands and can be bilateral. It has been noted that pain increases with eating, and the disease process goes into cycles of remission alternating with exacerbation. Usually, the gland is diffusely enlarged and may resemble a neoplasm. It has been associated at times with bulimia and ductal obstruction with secondary inflammatory reaction. Fine needle aspiration usually produces bloody smears with few cells. However, occasionally the aspirates would be cellular where mucous, proteinaceous material may be observed in the background with occasional acini surrounded by chronic inflammatory cells and occasional atrophy and squamous metaplasia (Figures 4.4 and 4.5). If the gland is removed, then the histological sections will show similar features (Figure 4.6). The differential diagnosis includes mucocele and low-grade mucoepidermoid carcinoma. On the one hand, mucocele has a characteristic clinical picture, and the aspirates would be hypocellular and sometimes contain macrophages. On the other hand, low-grade mucoepi-dermoid carcinoma aspirate smears usually yield mucous cells and a mixture of intermediate and myoepithelial cells. Aspirates that contain many lymphoid cells, monotony, and lymphoid cells with atypia raise the possibility of lymphoproliferative disorders, which needs immunophenotypic analysis to make the distinction.

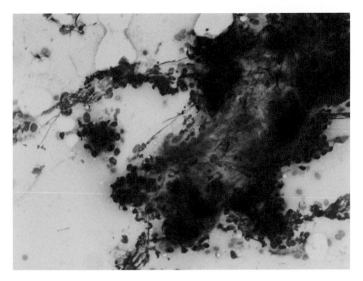

FIGURE 4.4. Salivary gland acini are seen with crushing, cellular debris and surrounded by lymphocytes characteristic of chronic sialadenitis (Diff Quik stain, 400×).

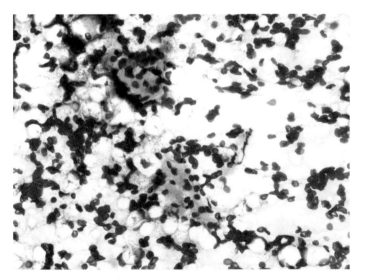

FIGURE 4.5. Residual acini are observed surrounded by lymphocytes (Papanicolaou stain, 400×).

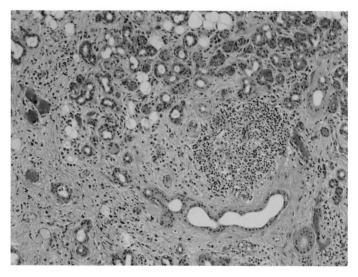

FIGURE 4.6. Representative histological section from a case of chronic sialadenitis showing chronic inflammation in the form of follicle and intervening fibrosis (hematoxylin and eosin stain, 200×).

4.6   ACUTE VIRAL PAROTITIS (MUMPS)

Mumps was the classic childhood infection. It spread by droplet or by direct spread from oropharyngeal secretions that contain the paramyxovirus. The clinical disease only manifests in 60% to 70% of those who are exposed. Universal immunization, which began in 1977, has made the clinical disease unusual in developed countries. Occasional outbreaks were observed mostly in teenagers or patients who were in their 20s and who did not receive the second dose of their vaccine.

The disease is characterized by grossly enlarged and modestly tender parotid glands. Mumps is a benign disease in most cases but may be complicated by meningoencephalitis, pancreatitis, orchitis, or deafness. The treatment of the disease is supportive and symptomatic. Fine needle aspiration for diagnostic purposes in cases of mumps parotitis is not indicated. It is worthwhile to mention that viral parotitis has also been reported to be caused by other viruses, such as influenza virus, parainfluenza virus, and HIV.

4.7   HIV SIALADENITIS/PAROTITIS

HIV parotitis occurs in children far more often than in adults who are HIV positive. The gland in those affected is firm, nontender, and chronically enlarged. Usually few or no symptoms are present. A parotid cyst or lymphadenopathy may be the presenting complaint in patients with HIV infection. Currently, it is wise to test for HIV infection in any patient who presents with enlarged or cystic parotid gland. Fine needle aspiration reveals benign lymphoepithelial lesion (BLL) in the form of a mixture of salivary gland cells (acini, epithelial, and myoepithelial cells) in a background of mixed (polymorphous) lymphoid cell population. These lesions have been described commonly as LESA. Features similar to benign lymphoid hyperplasia sometimes can dominate where the aspirates contain lymphoglandular bodies and tingible body macrophages. The pathogenesis is thought to be secondary to ductal obstruction by lymphoid hyperplasia. Usually, an HIV-associated parotid cysts are multiple and/or bilateral. Fine needle aspiration of these cysts shows clear to turbid fluid but may appear milky or purulent. The inflammatory cells are polymorphous and include macrophages and mixed lymphoid cells, with follicular center cell immunoblasts, histocytes, hemosiderin laden macrophages, and rarely, epithelial cells. In rare occasions, squamous metaplastic cells can be observed. The differential diagnosis of these lesions includes lymphoproliferative disorders in which immunophenotyping would be critical to make the distinction. In cases where squamous cells are present, squamous cell carcinoma should be ruled out. In the latter, the squamous cells would be atypical, and they may represent either high-grade mucoepidermoid carcinoma or metastatic squamous cell carcinoma from a head and neck primary.

4.8   TUBERCULOUS SIALADENITIS/PAROTITIS

Mycobacterial tuberculosis is an uncommon cause of parotitis. In the past, nontuberculous mycobacteria species were the most common cause of parotitis. The incidence of mycobacteria tuberculosis parotitis has been increasing. Fine needle aspiration of the infected parotid gland would show necrotizing granulomas. Sometimes, these granulomas are poorly formed and may be few in number in a background of necrosis. A careful search for acid fast bacilli on cell block material may clinch the diagnosis long before the culture which takes weeks and may be difficult. Sometimes immediate and quick diagnosis can be achieved by utilizing mycobacterial polymerase chain reaction (PCR) on the aspirated material. The parotid glands return to normal in 1 to 3 months after treatment. Untreated cases may progress to a draining fistula and fibrosis.

4.9   OTHER GRANULOMATOUS SIALADENITIS

Granulomatous sialadenitis has also been reported in sarcoidosis, cat scratch disease, toxins, and a variety of fungal infections. Lymph node involvement is

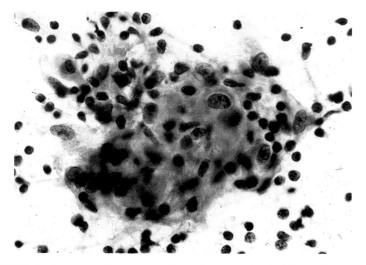

FIGURE 4.7. Aspirate smear from a case of granulomatous sialadenitis showing a granuloma with no evidence of necrosis. The patient was found to have sarcoidosis after excluding other etiologies (Papanicolaou stain, 400×).

more common than glandular involvement in these cases. Fine needle aspiration reveals granulomatous inflammation where it is characteristically non-necrotizing in sarcoidosis and the granulomas are well defined (Figures 4.7 and 4.8). Sarcoidosis mostly affects the African American population in the age group of 20 to 40 years. Although, non-necrotizing granulomatous sialadenitis is characteristic, sarcoidosis is a diagnosis of exclusion. Heerfordt–Waldenström syndrome consists of the combination of sarcoidosis with involvement of parotid glands, fever, anterior uvietis, and facial palsy. When this syndrome is diagnosed, treatment with systemic steroids is indicated.

4.10 NECROTIZING SIALOMETAPLASIA

Necrotizing sialometaplasia is an uncommon, benign disease process that can mimic cancer. It rarely affects the major glands, whereas the palatine small salivary glands are most commonly involved. A mass lesion with associated ulceration at the junction of hard–soft palate adjacent to midline is characteristic. Making this diagnosis by FNAB is difficult. Usually, the diagnosis is confirmed by histological examination of a biopsy. The histological features exhibit severe chronic inflammation associated with extensive squamous metaplasia of the ducts and occasionally fragments of granulation tissue. To rule out mucoepidermoid carcinoma or squamous cell carcinoma, a thorough search for prominent cytological and nuclear atypia is helpful.

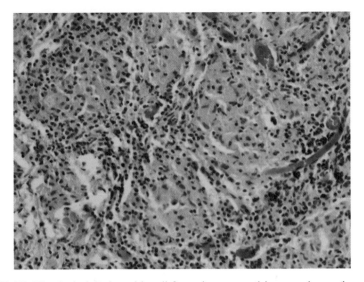

FIGURE 4.8. Histological section with well-formed non-necrotizing granulomas characteristic of Sarcoidosis of salivary gland similar to what is seen in the cytological smears (hematoxylin and eosin stain, 200×).

4.11 AUTOIMMUNE SIALADENITIS

Autoimmune sialadenitis used to be known as Mikulicz disease, but currently Sjögren syndrome is a common term used. Mikulicz disease was an older term used to describe a painless swelling of the parotid or lacrimal glands. It was thought to be caused by a benign lymphoid epitheloid lesion. Usually, it is observed in middle-aged women, but it can affect any age. The involvement can be bilateral, diffuse, and/or cystic. However, solid enlargement has been reported. The disease can progress and lead to destruction of the salivary glands, which can ultimately cause sicca syndrome. FNABs are not usually indicated; however, in cases where solid enlargement is observed, the aspirates usually reveal nonspecific changes in the form of mixed inflammation and reactive cellular changes.

Hensik Sjögren was a Swedish ophthalmologist who in 1930 described a case of chronic parotitis associated with keratoconjunctivitis sicca. The disease most commonly occurs in people whose age group ranged from 40 to 60 years old. However, it was also observed to affect small children. The prevalence of this type of parotitis in a woman versus men is 9 to 1. The involved parotid gland is enlarged and tender at times. A benign lymphoepithelial lesion is the characteristic cytopathological finding that is difficult to differentiate from other inflammatory parotitis. The clinical data would be the deciding criteria to make the diagnosis of Sjögren syndrome. In 1953, Morgan and Castleman reported a massive lymphoid infiltration over the parotid gland with atrophy of the acini, proliferation of the cells of the small ducts, which led to a narrowing of the lumen, and finally an obliteration of the ducts. John Godwin, a New York pathologist, published a series of parotidectomy cases in 1952 with similar and overlapping features.

Currently, Sjögren syndrome encompasses all these conditions and is classified into three types: type I, II and III. Type I consists of keratoconjunctivitis sicca (dry mouth and dry eyes); type II consists of the aforementioned symptoms plus rheumatoid arthritis; and type III occurs when lymphoma supervenes. Serologically, antinuclear antibodies are present in 90% of the cases. Patients are usually at a higher risk of developing lymphoma (particularly B-cell non-Hodgkin's lymphoma) and carcinoma. FNABs show marked lymphocytic infiltrate of the salivary gland, whereas in other cases, the aspirate smears show features similar to what has been mentioned in LESA or BLL. If lymphoma has developed, then usually the aspirates yield more monotonous lymphoid cell population, and immunophenotypic analysis would be needed to confirm the diagnosis. Because of the increased risk of squamous cell carcinomas, a careful search for atypical large squamous cells is needed to exclude this possibility.

4.12   RADIATION SIALADENITIS

In postradiation treatments, patients may develop salivary gland enlargement, particularly the submandibular glands. Chronic radiation changes includes parenchymal atrophy, with ductal metaplasia, proliferation, fibrosis, and dilatation. When FNAB is performed, the glands are usually hypocellular. Occasionally, atypical epithelial cells would be present, which poses challenges to exclude neoplasia. In these circumstances, surgical excision would be needed to confirm the diagnosis. Therefore, extreme caution should be exercised when interpreting hypocellular smears of salivary glands with atypical cells in patients with history of radiation.

4.13   SIALADENOSIS (SIALOSIS)

Sialadenosis is a diffuse, usually bilateral, noninflammatory, non-neoplastic salivary gland enlargement (Figure 4.9). It can affect both glands. Sialadenosis may result in a chipmunk-like appearance. It is reported to be associated with autoimmune process, peripheral neuropathy, and metabolic derangement (i. e., alcoholics, malnutrition, diabetes, and drug induced). There is evidence of hypertrophy of the acinic cell with fatty infiltration, but there is no evidence of inflammation or neoplasm. Fine needle aspiration biopsy of this lesion can be painful, but when performed, the results reveal normal salivary gland components, and a careful evaluation may show larger than usual acini and acinic cells (Figures 4.10 and 4.11).

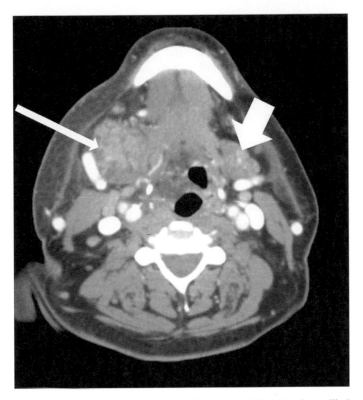

FIGURE 4.9. Computerized tomography image of a patient with right submandibular swelling found to be caused by sialosis through fine needle aspiration; see Figures 4.10 and 4.11. The long arrow points to the swollen right submandibular gland without any evidence of mass or infiltration to the surrounding structures with normal-appearing consistency similar to the left submandibular one (short arrow). The consistency and the size of the gland on the left side are within normal limits.

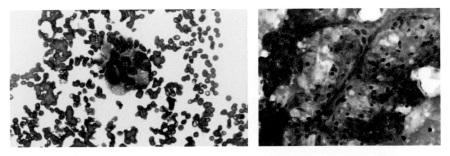

FIGURE 4.10. The smear on the left side shows enlarged acinus in sialosis compared with normal-sized acini on the right where the images are taken at the same magnification (Diff Quik stain, 600×).

4.14 SALIVARY GLAND CYST

Salivary gland cysts can appear at any age. Most are acquired and non-neoplastic, and they are either retention cysts or mucocele. These non-neoplastic cysts usually occur on the floor of the mouth or the lower lip. Fine needle aspirate biopsy usually obtains clear or cloudy fluid. Cytologically, the cyst fluid contains only a few cells, mostly macrophages and occasional degenerated (ghost cells) epithelial cells (Figure 4.12).

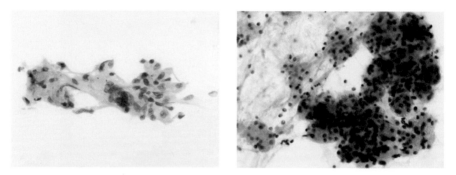

FIGURE 4.11. Smears from the same patient; the smear on the left side shows enlarged acini in sialosis compared with normal-sized acini on the right where the images are taken at the same magnification (Papanicolaou stain, 600×).

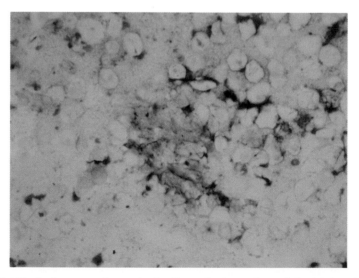

FIGURE 4.12. Aspirate smear from a simple salivary gland cyst where cellular debris and ghost of epithelial cells in a background of proteinaceous material are observed (Papanicolaou stain, 600×).

Congenital cysts can occur in the parotid gland representing a branchial cleft anomaly. In rare circumstances, a dermoid cyst (mature cystic teratoma) can affect salivary glands where FNAB may show different types of epithelial cells and sometimes hair elements. When suspected, these lesions must be excised.

RECOMMENDED READINGS

Aggarwal AP, Jayaram G, Mandal AK. Sarcoidosis diagnosed on fine-needle aspiration cytology of salivary glands: a report of three cases. Diagn Cytopathol 1989;5:289–292.

Carlson ER. Diagnosis and management of salivary gland infections. Oral Maxillofac Surg Clin N Am 2009;21:293–312.

Cascarini L, McGurk M. Epidemiology of salivary gland infections. Oral Maxillofac Surg Clin N Am 2009;21:353–357.

Droese M. Cytological diagnosis of sialadenosis, sialadenitis, and parotid cysts by fine-needle aspiration biopsy. Adv Otorhinolaryngol 1981;26:49–96.

Harris NL. Lymphoid proliferations of the salivary glands. Am J Clin Pathol 1999;111:S94–103.

Henry-Stanley MJ, Beneke J, Bardales RH, Stanley MW. Fine needle aspiration of normal tissue from enlarged salivary glands: sialosis or missed target? Diagn Cytopathol 1995;13:300–303.

Kreisel FH, Frater JL, Hassan A, El-Mofty SK. Cystic lymphoid hyperplasia of the parotid gland in HIV-positive and HIV-negative patients: quantitative immunopathology. Oral Surg Oral Med Oral Pathol Oral Radiol Endod 2010;109:567–574.

Schreiber A, Hershman G. Non-HIV viral infections of the salivary glands. Oral Maxillofac Surg Clin N Am 2009;21:331–338.

Wong DS, Wong LY. Cystic parotid swelling on FNA: significance on clinical management. Otolaryngol Head Neck Surg 2004;130:593–596.

CHAPTER 5

PLEOMORPHIC ADENOMA

JINING FENG, MD, PHD and MOUSA A. AL-ABBADI, MD, FIAC

5.1 INTRODUCTION

Pleomorphic adenoma, which is also known as mixed tumor, is a benign tumor composed of a variable mixture of benign epithelial and myoepithelial cells with a stromal background composed of a mucoid, myxoid, or chondroid look.

5.2 CLINICAL FEATURES

Pleomorphic adenoma (PA) is the most common neoplasm of all salivary glands in both adults and children. It represents approximately 65% of parotid tumors, 50% of submandibular tumors, and 40% of all minor salivary tumors. A wide age distribution has been observed with an average age in the fourth decade of life. Women are affected more than men, with a female-to-male ratio of approximately 2:1. The most common site is the parotid gland, and most tumors are located in the superficial lobe. The submandibular gland and palate are the second most common sites but are six to seven times less likely than the parotid gland. Clinically, it presents commonly as a slow-growing, firm, painless mass. A computed tomography (CT) scan usually shows a well-circumscribed tumor with lobulation. The radiological appearance of the cut surface of the tumor can be heterogeneous depending on the different proportions of its components. If the tumor is not well delineated on CT scan, then magnetic resonance imaging can be more helpful. A lobulated contour with a low signal capsule on T2-weighted images is able to characterize most PAs. Fine needle aspiration biopsy is often used for preoperative diagnosis.

Salivary Gland Cytology: A Color Atlas, Edited by Mousa A. Al-Abbadi
Copyright © 2011 Wiley-Blackwell

Rarely, synchronous tumors besides PA on the same side or the other side with same or different histological type occur. PA, Warthin's tumor, myoepithelioma, salivary duct carcinoma, and mucoepidermoid carcinoma have been reported. However, the most common tumor that can be present in association with PA is a Warthin's tumor.

5.3 CYTOLOGIC FEATURES AND HISTOLOGIC CORRELATES

The aspirate smears of PA contain a mixture of epithelial cells, myoepithelial cells, and stromal matrix components. The epithelial cells are small to moderately sized cuboidal cells with distinct cell border and bland nuclear features arranged in cohesive sheets, clusters, or single cells (Figures 5.1 and 5.2). The myoepithelial cells may have a spindled, plasmacytoid, clear cell, or epithelioid appearance, and they are often found within the stromal myxoid matrix material, in loose clusters, or individually (Figures 5.3 and 5.4). One of the most characteristic features of PA is the fibrillary chondromyxoid matrix material, which appears as an intense magenta color on air-dried Diff-Quik stain (Figure 5.5) and as a pale green gray color on Papanicolaou stain (Figure 5.6). This matrix material has fibrillary ragged edges, often with embedded myoepithelial cells (Figure 5.7). Table 5.1 summarizes the key cytologic features. The proportion of each element can vary considerably from case to case. In some patients, the epithelial element predominates,

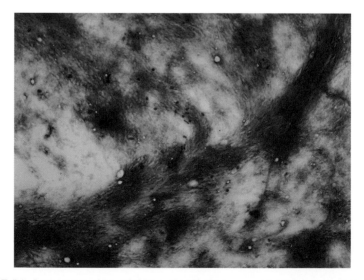

FIGURE 5.1. Low-power view exhibiting the fibrillary myxoid background that appears magenta red on Diff-Quik stain. Embedded are scattered myoepithelial cells (Diff-Quik stain, 200×).

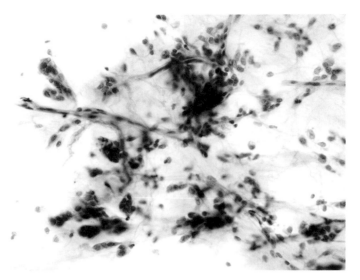

FIGURE 5.2. A high-power view of the fibrillary myxoid stroma with embedded myoepithelial cells (Papanicolaou stain, 400×).

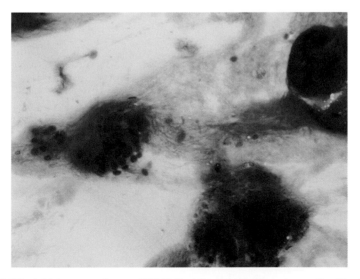

FIGURE 5.3. A high-power view on Diff-Quik stain with fibrillary stroma, few bland naked nuclei of myoepithelial cells, and few epithelial cells (left side of the image) with a suggestion of an acinus (Diff-Quik stain, 400×).

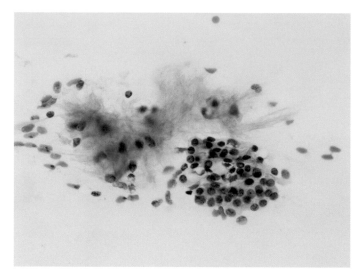

FIGURE 5.4. A high-power view with all three elements: fibrillary stroma, myoepithelial cells, and epithelial cells. The myoepithelial cells are embedded in the stroma, and their nuclei are slightly spindle. The epithelial cells form acini with basally located bland nuclei and small nucleoli (Papanicolaou stain, 600×).

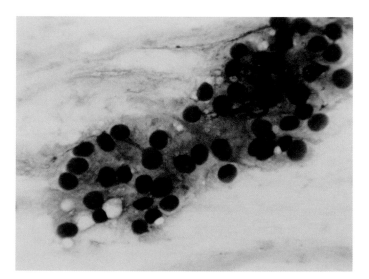

FIGURE 5.5. High-power view of epithelial cells forming acini with bland basally located nuclei (Diff-Quik stain, 1,000× oil).

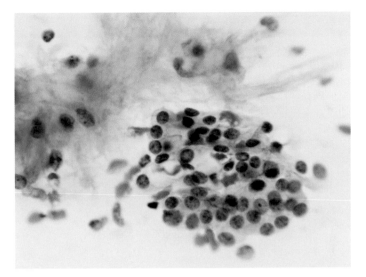

FIGURE 5.6. Another high-power view with all three elements exhibiting similar features (Papanicolaou stain, 1,000× oil).

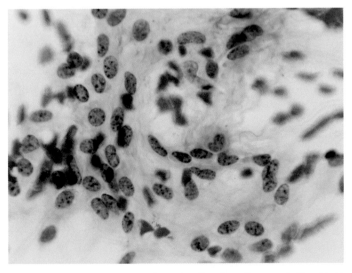

FIGURE 5.7. High-power view of myoepithelial cells. The cells are spindle with bland nuclei and inconspicuous nucleoli (Papanicolaou stain, 1,000× oil).

TABLE 5.1. Key diagnostic features of PA

- Mixture of epithelial and mesenchymal components
- Fibrillary chondromyxoid matrix, often embedded with myoepithelial cells
- Epithelial cells in sheets, ducts, or singly with distinct cytoplasmic border and bland cellular and nuclear features
- Myoepithelial cells; can be plasmacytoid, spindle shaped, or clear but all with bland nuclei

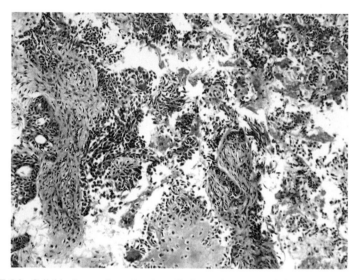

FIGURE 5.8. Cell block correlate showing all three elements and their benign appearance (hematoxylin and eosin stain, 100×).

whereas others are richer in chondromyxoid stroma. Crystalloids such as tyrosine-rich and oxalate crystals, squamous or oncocytic metaplasia, and mucin production can be observed in some cases.

It is usually not difficult to make the diagnosis of PAs if the lesion is sampled adequately and classic cytologic features are present. However, in a small percentage of cases, some features such as cellular aspirates with scant matrix, cytologic atypia, squamous metaplasia, and mucin production may pose difficulties.

The histological sections of PA also can be variable depending on the proportions of its components. However, usually the basic three elements exist and the key features are well circumscribed mostly with a capsule, bland cellular and nuclear features, and rarity of mitosis (Figure 5.8). The epithelial cells vary and can exhibit diversity in their size and shape; however, they are bland and lack cytological atypia. The stromal properties also can vary and range from soft chondromyxoid and sometimes mucoid, hard fibrocartilagenous, bony, and occasionally lipofibromatous.

5.4 CYTOLOGIC DIFFERENTIAL DIAGNOSIS

Richly cellular aspirates with scant matrix material may preclude a definitive diagnosis of PA. The main differential diagnoses include basal cell adenoma and adenoid cystic carcinoma. A distinction between PA and basal cell adenoma is not important because there is no clinical significance in terms of management to make the distinction between these two diagnoses. In general, PA contains a greater amount of stroma with a fibrillary appearance, and basal cell adenoma has thick hyaline bands around cell clusters. Occasionally, well-demarcated hyaline globules resembling a thick basement membrane material of adenoid cystic carcinoma are found in otherwise typical PAs. Adequate sampling of the lesion is important as well as attention to cytologic details of epithelial/myoepithelial cells. The epithelial cells of PA have well-defined cytoplasm and a bland nuclear chromatin, whereas adenoid cystic carcinoma has scanty cytoplasm with greater nuclear hyperchromasia and coarseness (more basaloid). When it is difficult to resolve, proper differential diagnoses is recommended.

Squamous metaplasia (Figure 5.9) and mucin (Figure 5.10) production is sometimes found in PA, which might suggest mucoepidermoid carcinoma or squamous cell carcinoma. Searching for typical features of PA, including the absence of mucin-producing epithelial cells and intermediate cells makes

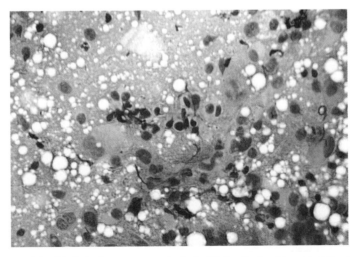

FIGURE 5.9. PA with foci of squamous metaplasia. Notice the hard (squamoid) cytoplasm of these cells. In other fields, all the classic features of PA were present (May–Grünwald–Giemsa [MGG] stain, 400×).

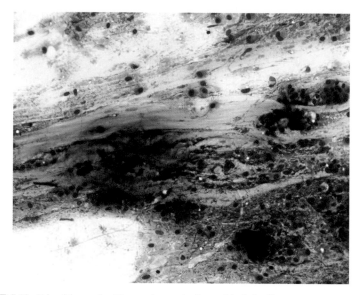

FIGURE 5.10. PA with mucin. No mucin-producing epithelial cells were present, and all the classic features of PA were present in other fields (MGG, 400×).

mucoepidermoid carcinoma less likely. However, low-grade mucoepidermoid carcinoma can be misdiagnosed as PA (or vice versa) because its mucinous material can be mistaken as myxoid stroma (especially with the Papanicolaou stain), and the intermediate cells are misinterpreted as epithelial/myoepithelial cells of PA. Similarly, oncocytic metaplasia can sometimes occur in association with PA (Figures 5.11 and 5.12). Although this change is not common, it can occur where sampling will be critical to make the correct diagnosis. If the needle hits only the oncocytic area, then misdiagnosis as Warthin's tumor may occur. Again, using appropriate sampling technique and confirming the presence of classic PA features in other areas or slides of the smears will ensure a correct diagnosis. Cytologic atypia can be observed in PAs and is usually mild to moderate and focal. However, when severe cytologic atypia including nuclear enlargement, abnormal nuclear chromatin, and prominent nucleoli is present, especially when associated with necrosis or mitoses, then carcinoma ex-PA might be possible. In addition, the presence of long-standing tumor mass with recent quick enlargement is a good clinical clue. Occasionally, PA aspirates exhibit rich myoepithelial cells, which suggests pure myoepithelioma. Good sampling and search for epithelial cells and the associated chondromyxoid stroma serve as a clue to make the distinction. In cases where these two elements are scarce or difficult to find, a diagnosis of benign myoepithelial-cell-rich neoplasm with a comment explaining the differential diagnosis is justified and is a reasonable approach.

Rarely, a benign-appearing mixed tumor of the salivary gland metastasizes to the lung, bone, or other organs, and they are called benign metastasizing

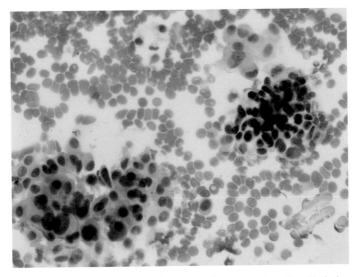

FIGURE 5.11. Smears of PA with oncocytic metaplasia; the smaller cells with darker nuclei are myoepithelial cells, and the other groups with larger cells and more ample cytoplasm are the cells with oncocytic metaplasia (Papanicolaou stain, 400×).

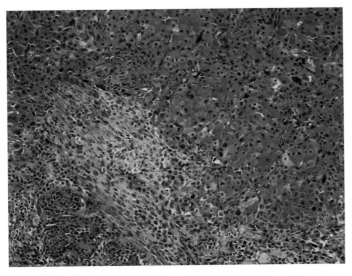

FIGURE 5.12. The histological correlate of the previous smear (Figure 5.11). The section showed oncocytic metaplasia on the right half and adjacent classic PA on the left half (hematoxylin and eosin stain, 200×).

mixed tumors. These tumors have the typical features of PA without malignant cytologic features. A distinction between these two by cytologic examination is almost impossible, although some have reported mild nuclear atypia found in a benign metastazing mixed tumor. Multiple local recurrences of benign appearing mixed tumor may raise suspicion of this rare entity. Table 5.2 summarizes the differential diagnosis and provides clues to make the distinction.

TABLE 5.2.	
Major differential diagnosis of PA	Clues to make the distinction
Adenoid cystic carcinoma	Adenoid cystic carcinoma usually exhibits globules and cylinders of a cellular pink basement membrane material with sharp borders surrounded by basaloid cells. The cells have greater nuclear hyperchromasia and the chromatin is coarse. PA may occasionally have well-demarcated hyaline globules, but they are focal in otherwise typical PA fibrillary matrix. The epithelial/myoepithelial cells are bland.
Low grade mucoepidermoid carcinoma	Low-grade mucoepidermoid carcinoma contains abundant extracellular mucin plus mucus cells, intermediate cells, and epidermoid cells. PA may have squamous metaplasia, mucin production, and cystic degeneration in otherwise typical PA. The key is a high index of suspicion and searching for typical features of both tumors.
Carcinoma ex PA	Malignant mixed tumor has large numbers of severe atypical cells with nuclear enlargement and prominent nucleoli. Necrosis and mitoses may be observed. Cytologic atypia in some PAs is usually mild to moderate and focal. If cytologic atypia is worrisome, a diagnosis of PA with atypia is sometimes warranted.
Chronic sialadenitis	Chronic inflammatory conditions may present as a mass-like lesion. Usually, aspirates are sparsely cellular-containing epithelial cell aggregates and fibrous stroma. Inflammatory cells may be found. The stroma is not that intensely stained on Diff-Quik stain and it is not fibrillary in nature. Sialadenitis lacks epithelial tumor cell clusters but may contain scattered essentially normal acini.
Warthin's tumor	Warthin's tumor has oncocytic epithelium with a background of lymphocytes. PA with oncocytic metaplasia will also have myoepithelial cells and fibrillary chondromyxoid stroma.
Myoepithelioma	Myoepithelioma lacks epithelial and chondromyxoid matrix elements.

5.5   TREATMENT AND PROGNOSIS

Surgical excision with a margin of normal tissue or superficial parotidectomy is the treatment of choice for PA. In most instances excision is curative; however, recurrence can occur, with a range of incidence between 0% and 8%. Recurrence is usually a result of incomplete surgical removal because of the occasional pod-like tumor projections into surrounding normal gland. Malignancy can occur in 5% to 10% of long-standing PA and may occur long after the initial excision.

RECOMMENDED READINGS

Curry JL, Petruzzelli GJ, McClatchey KD, Lingen MW. Synchronous benign and malignant salivary gland tumors in ipsilateral glands: a report of two cases and a review of literature. Head Neck 2002;24;301–306.

Bien S, Kaminski B, Kopcyznski J, Sygut J. The synchroneous tumors of different histopathology in the parotid glands. Otolaryngol Pol 2006;60:703–708.

Viguer JM, Vicandi B, Jiménez-Heffernan JA, López-Ferrer P, Limeres MA. Fine needle aspiration cytology of pleomorphic adenoma. An analysis of 212 cases. Acta Cytol 1997;41:786–794.

Kapadia SB, Dusenbery D, Dekker A. Fine needle aspiration of pleomorphic adenoma and adenoid cystic carcinoma of salivary gland origin. Acta Cytol 1997;41:487–492.

Lee SS, Cho KJ, Jang JJ, Ham EK. Differential diagnosis of adenoid cystic carcinoma from pleomorphic adenoma of the salivary gland on fine needle aspiration cytology. Acta Cytol 1996;40:1246–52.

Brachtel EF, Pilch BZ, Khettry U, Zembowicz A, Faquin WC. Fine-needle aspiration biopsy of a cystic pleomorphic adenoma with extensive adnexa-like differentiation: differential diagnostic pitfall with mucoepidermoid carcinoma. Diagn Cytopathol 2003;28:100–103.

Nigam S, Kumar N, Jain S. Cytomorphologic spectrum of carcinoma ex pleomorphic adenoma. Acta Cytol 2004;48:309–314.

Manucha V, Ioffe OB. Metastasizing pleomorphic adenoma of the salivary gland. Arch Pathol Lab Med 2008;132:1445–1447.

Benign metastasizing pleomorphic adenoma of salivary gland: diagnosis of bone lesions by fine-needle aspiration biopsy. Diagn Cytopathol 1992;8:384–937.

Zhang S, Bao R, Bagby J, Abreo F. Fine needle aspiration of salivary glands: 5-year experience from a single academic center. Acta Cytol 2009;53:375–382.

CHAPTER 6

WARTHIN'S TUMOR

MOUSA A. AL-ABBADI, MD, FIAC

6.1 INTRODUCTION

Warthin's tumor (WT) is considered a benign primary parotid gland neoplasm, which is composed of a mixture of oncocytic cells, basal cells, and stroma that contains numerous lymphocytes. Usually, the mixture is arranged in papillary and cystic structures.

6.2 CLINICAL FEATURES

The tumor involves the parotid gland almost exclusively and sometimes the intraparotid and periparotid lymph nodes. It is the second most common primary salivary gland tumor preceded only by pleomorphic adenoma. It comprises approximately 4% and up to 30% of all epithelial salivary gland tumors. Geographical variations have been reported. The tumor occurs most commonly after the age of 40 years with a mean age around the sixth decade. It is known to be more common in Caucasians and Asians than in African Americans. A strong association between cigarette smoking and Warthin's tumor is well known, but the exact mechanism is unclear. An additional association was reported with history of radiation and pre-existing auto-immune diseases. With the increasing numbers of female smokers in the recent decades, the previously male predilection is now much weaker. WT is a salivary tumor that can be multicentric and is commonly bilateral. The most common presentation is painless mass or swelling of variable duration. Pain or facial paralysis are rare and occur when associated significant

Salivary Gland Cytology: A Color Atlas, Edited by Mousa A. Al-Abbadi
Copyright © 2011 Wiley-Blackwell

inflammation and fibrosis are present. Radiologically, WT is characteristically well circumscribed, partially cystic, and exhibits strong enhancement.

6.3   CYTOPATHOLOGICAL FEATURES

While aspirating a WT and because of the cystic nature of the lesion, sometimes a dirty, dark brown, thick fluid (it has been commonly described in the literature as machine-oil-like content) can be observed. The aspirate smears characteristically contain numerous lymphocytes admixed with epithelial oncocytic cells and a protein-rich background. The background can be appreciated easily on Diff-Quik stain. The lymphocytes are small and appear mature and more commonly monotonous in nature. The epithelial cells are large and polygonal, and they exhibit an abundant, slightly granular cytoplasm. Usually, they are arranged in two-dimensional sheets (Figure 6.1) rather than three-dimensional groups, and occasionally they form papillae. The granular cytoplasm is more evident on Diff-Quik stain (Figure 6.2) where it is deep blue, and it appears grayish blue on the Papanicolaou stain (Figure 6.3). The nuclei are round to occasionally ovoid and can be located centrally or eccentrically with evenly distributed chromatin (Figure 6.4). Small and occasionally larger nucleoli are present. Cell block stained with hematoxylin and eosin stain will recapitulate the features of cytological smears and the histological correlates (Figure 6.5). The oncocytic cells show their bright eosinophilic and granular cytoplasm, as well as the attached

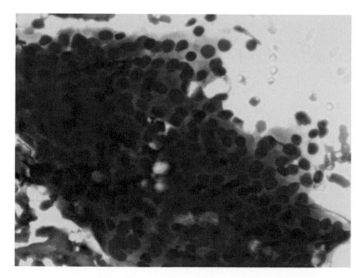

FIGURE 6.1. The cells are slightly large with abundant cytoplasm. The nuclei are bland (Diff Quik Stain 400×).

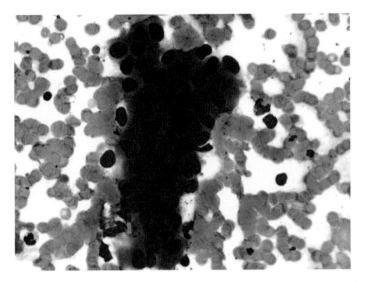

FIGURE 6.2. The cells are slightly large with abundant granular cytoplasm and the nuclei are bland. Some mature-appearing small lymphocytes are seen in the background (Diff-Quik stain, 600×).

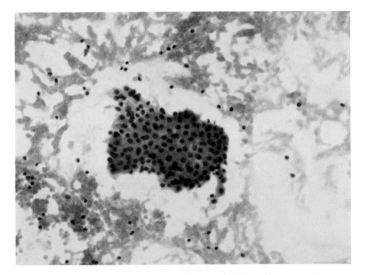

FIGURE 6.3. On Papanicolaou stain, the cells show similar features with the cytoplasm exhibiting blue-greenish color. The nuclei are bland and are located either centrally or peripherally. Numerous small lymphocytes are observed in the background (Papanicolaou stain, 200×).

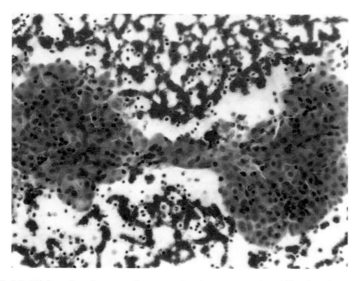

FIGURE 6.4. Higher view from another case showing more eosinophilic abundant cytoplasm and small bland nuclei. Numerous lymphocytes are observed in the background (Papanicolaou stain, 400×).

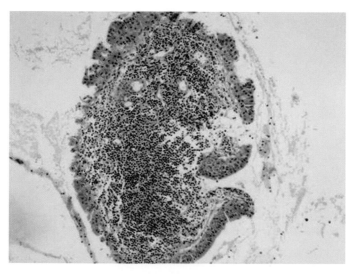

FIGURE 6.5. Cell block section showing both the benign oncocytic cells and numerous small lymphoid cells in the background (hematoxylin and eosin stain, 200×).

TABLE 6.1. The key cytological features of Warthin's tumor
Oncocytic cells in sheets of two dimensions
Numerous mature small lymphocytes
Dirty proteinaceous background

underlying lymphocytic rich stroma. Table 6.1 summarizes the key characteristic cytological features. Attention has to be paid for occasional
additional features that sometimes can be observed in WT cases, such as
squamous and mucinous metaplasia that will be translated to observing few
squamous and mucinous cells. The presence of these occasional cells raises
the possibility of mucoepidermoid carcinoma and metastatic squamous cell
carcinoma. However, identifying the previously mentioned components and
the lack of cytological atypia help to support the diagnosis of WT. The other
differential is oncocytoma and acinic cell carcinoma. These two neoplasms
will not have the additional two components: lymphocytes and the proteinaceous background In addition, oncocytomas are usually solid and not
cystic. Therefore, the presence of cystic tumor areas with oncocytes always
supports WT diagnosis. Although rare, the presence of both pleomorphic
adenoma and WT can occur in the parotid gland; in these cases, good
sampling will yield features of both. One safe approach is to raise the
possibility when facing an aspirate with lymphocytes, oncocytes, and myxoid
fibrillary background. Table 6.2 summarizes the differential diagnosis and
demonstrates clues to help make the distinctions. Spontaneous and fine needle
aspiration (FNA)-induced partial or complete infarction can sometimes occur in
WT; such tumors will yield mainly necrotic material and cellular debris, which
makes it difficult to establish the diagnosis.

6.4   HISTOLOGICAL CORRELATES

On gross evaluation, WT is at least partially cystic and well circumscribed
ovoid or round. The cut surface usually shows slit-like cystic spaces with
mucoid, tan, or brown thick fluid (which is described as machinery oil
material). The classic histological features are summarized rightfully by the
old name "papillary cystadenoma lymphomatosum." The sections show a
cystic and papillary tumor lined by two layers of benign and bland-appearing
epithelium, an oncocytic component with abundant eosinophilic cytoplasm,
and another basal layer with smaller cells. The cystic spaces contain benign
small lymphoid cells that sometimes form lymphoid follicles. Immunopheno-
typically, the lymphocytes are polyclonal T cells in nature.

TABLE 6.2. Differential diagnosis of WT and clues to make the distinction

Pleomorphic adenoma with oncocytic metaplasia	WT lacks the fibrillary mayxoid matrix background, and pleomorphic adenoma will not have the combination of oncocytic cells and the mature small lymphoid cellular background.
Mucoepidermoid carcinoma (MEC), low grade	MEC lacks the combination of oncocytic cells and the mature small lymphoid cellular background, and WT will not have mucinous cells or mucoid background.
MEC, high grade	MEC lacks the combination of oncocytic cells and the mature small lymphoid cellular background, and WT will lack mucinous cells, significant cytological atypia, atypical squamous cells, and necrosis.
Oncocytoma and oncocytic carcinoma	Oncocytoma will contain pure oncocytic cell population, and if malignant, it will show in addition significant cytological and nuclear atypia and necrosis. They are never cystic. WT will contain a combination of oncocytic cells and the mature small lymphoid cellular background.* The Oncocytes on both categories are similar.
Acinic cell carcinoma	The smears of acinic cell carcinoma are usually more cellular; the cytoplasm is less granular and the nucleus is more uniform and smaller. The cytoplasmic granules of acinic cell carcinoma are Periodic acid Schiff stain positive and diastase resistant (PAS-D). While Phosphotungstic acid-hematoxylin (PTAH) will stain WT cytoplasm. However, good cell block will resolve the differential without special stain.
Lymphoma (this, in particular, includes the well-differentiated small cell size lymphomas, such as small lymphocytic lymphoma, MALT lymphoma, follicular lymphoma, and mantle cell lymphoma)	Lymphomas lack the oncocytic cells, and if the lymphoma arises from inside the salivary gland, then immunophenotyping using flow cytometry and/or immunohistochemistry on cell block material will be needed.

*Occasionally, WT may be lymphocyte poor; a good sampling technique will resolve the issue.

6.5 PROGNOSIS AND TREATMENT

Usually, WT is cured by surgical excision or enucleation, after which the recurrence rate is less than 5% and is caused mainly by multicentricity. Association with other salivary gland tumors is common in WT, and specifically pleomorphic adenoma can occur. Other rare associations that have been reported, including lymphoma and squamous cell carcinoma.

RECOMMENDED READINGS

Ballo MS, Shin HJ, Sneige N. Sources of diagnostic error in the fine-needle aspiration diagnosis of Warthin's tumor and clues to a correct diagnosis. Diagn Cytopathol 1997;17:230–234.

Barnes L, Eveson J, Reichart P, Sidransky D. Pathology & Genetics, Head and Tumours. World Health Organization Classification of Tumor Series. Lyon, France: IARC Press; 2005. p 263–265.

Cardoso SV, do Nascimento Souza KC, de Faria PR, Lima RA, Nascimento MF, Eisenberg AL, Dias FL, Loyola AM. Warthin's tumor at the Brazilian National Cancer Institute: additional evidence of homogeneous sex prevalence and association with other neoplasms. ORL J Otorhinolaryngol Relat Spec 2008;70:339–343.

Das DK, Petkar MA, Al-Mane NM, Sheikh ZA, Mallik MK, Anim JT. Role of fine needle aspiration cytology in the diagnosis of swellings in the salivary gland regions: a study of 712 cases. Med Princ Pract 2004;13:95–106.

Elagoz S, Gulluoglu M, Yilmazbayhan D, Ozer H, Arslan I. The value of fine-needle aspiration cytology in salivary gland lesions, 1994–2004. ORL J Otorhinolaryngol Relat Spec 2007;69:51–56.

Flezar M, Pogacnik A. Warthin's tumour: unusual vs. common morphological findings in fine needle aspiration biopsies. Cytopathology 2002;13:232–241.

Paulino AF, Huvos AG. Oncocytic and oncocytoid tumors of the salivary glands. Semin Diagn Pathol 1999;16:98–104.

Shikhani AH, Shikhani LT, Kuhajda FP, Allam CK. Warthin's tumor-associated neoplasms: report of two cases and review of the literature. Ear Nose Throat J 1993;72:264–269, 272–273.

Stewart CJ, MacKenzie K, McGarry GW, Mowat A. Fine-needle aspiration cytology of salivary gland: a review of 341 cases. Diagn Cytopathol 2000;22:139–146.

Verma K, Kapila K. Salivary gland tumors with a prominent oncocytic component. Cytologic findings and differential diagnosis of oncocytomas and Warthin's tumor on fine needle aspirates. Acta Cytol 2003;47:221–226.

CHAPTER 7

MUCOEPIDERMOID CARCINOMA

RUBA HALLOUSH, MD

7.1 INTRODUCTION

Mucoepidermoid carcinoma is a malignant epithelial neoplasm, composed of varying proportions of mucous, intermediate and epidermoid cells.

7.2 CLINICAL FEATURES

Mucoepidermoid carcinoma (MEC) is the most common primary salivary gland malignant tumor in adults and children and is the most common malignancy in the major and minor salivary glands. It comprises approximately 5% to 10% of all salivary gland tumors. It represents 22% of the malignant tumors in the major salivary glands and 41% in the minor salivary glands. MEC has a wide age range distribution, with a mean age of 45 years. Palate tumors tend to occur at a younger age. The male:female ratio is 2:3. Radiation has been implicated as a possible risk factor.

The parotid gland is involved most often, and it accounts for 45% of cases. The most common minor salivary glands affected are in the palate and buccal mucosa.

Clinical features depend on the grade of the tumor; usually, low-grade tumors are slow growing, cystic, and present as a painless mass with a 5-year survival rate of approximately 98%. High-grade tumors grow fast and have a high risk for lymph node and distant metastasis, as well as local recurrence. The 5-year survival rate is approximately 56%. Other symptoms include pain and facial nerve palsy. Radiologically, the appearance varies according to the grade; in addition, MEC can mimic other tumors in their radiologic appearance, and it should always be considered in the differential diagnosis. Low-grade tumors

Salivary Gland Cytology: A Color Atlas, Edited by Mousa A. Al-Abbadi
Copyright © 2011 Wiley-Blackwell

are well-circumscribed tumors that are enhanced with heterogeneous cystic component on computed tomography (CT) scan. The differential diagnosis includes pleomorphic adenoma and Warthin's tumor. However, high-grade tumors appear as an infiltrating, poorly defined, enhancing mass on CT scan. The differential diagnosis includes adenoid cystic carcinoma and other less common high-grade primary carcinomas, lymphoma and metastasis.

7.3   CYTOLOGICAL FEATURES

On histological grounds, MEC is graded into low, intermediate, and high grades. This division depends on multiple histological parameters that include the presence of cystic spaces, cellular differentiation, proportion of mucous cells, growth pattern, type of invasion, and cytological atypia. However, the application of three-tier grading system on cytological smears is difficult and cannot be reproducible. Therefore, cytological diagnosis by fine needle aspiration (FNA) usually is classified into low- and high-grade MEC. The hallmark for MEC diagnosis by FNA is the presence of a variable mixture of the three-cell components, which includes mucinous, squamoid, and intermediate cells. In low-grade tumors, extracellular mucin can be found in the background. It stains pale purple with the modified Romanowsky (Diff-Quik) stain and pale blue green with Papanicolaou stain (Figure 7.1). The cellular components are observed as groups and clusters, sometimes with identifiable transition from intermediate to mucinous cells (Figures 7.2 and 7.3). The intermediate cells

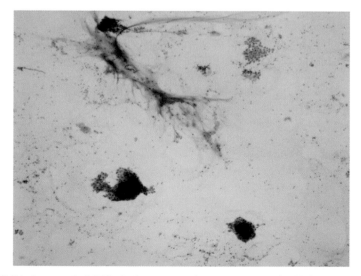

FIGURE 7.1. Low-grade MEC. At low power, there are groups of cells in a myxoid background. The mucin appears as pale, greenish blue on Papanicolaou stain (40×).

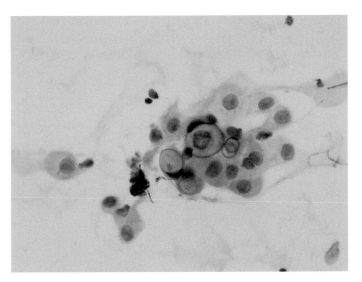

FIGURE 7.2. Low-grade MEC. At high power, this cluster contains both squamoid cells with well-defined hard cytoplasm and mucinous cells with vacuoles of mucin (400×).

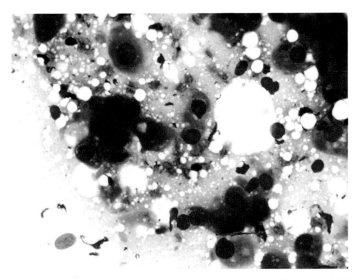

FIGURE 7.3. Low-grade MEC. Diff-Quik stain shows scattered cells, some with hard cytoplasm and some with vacuolated cytoplasm (400×).

resemble metaplastic cells and have a moderate amount of cytoplasm and round small nuclei. Mucinous cells have abundant vacuolated cytoplasm and may be columnar or signet-ring shaped. Squamoid cells have dense cytoplasm and polygonal shape. Usually, the mucinous cells predominate in low-grade tumors. Occasionally, one may observe clear and oncocytic cells mixed with these mucinous cells. The degree of cellular and nuclear atypia in low-grade MEC is minimal, and the aspirate smears lack tumor diathesis.

Aspirates from high-grade tumors show groups of cells with obvious malignant features including nuclear pleomorphism, hyperchromasia, clumped chromatin and prominent nucleoli (Figures 7.4 and 7.5). Mucinous cells are scarce compared with the squamoid and intermediate cells. In addition, it is common to view tumor diathesis in the background.

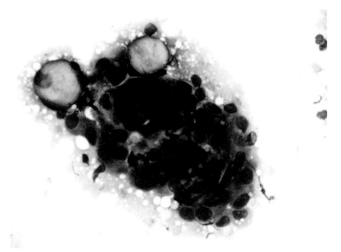

FIGURE 7.4. High grade mucoepidermoid carcinoma. Diff-Quik stain showing a three dimensional group of overlapping cells with few mucin containing cells (400×).

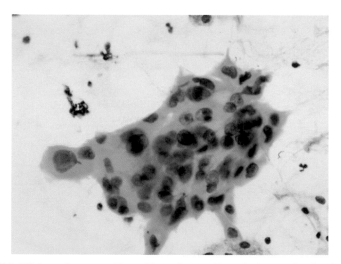

FIGURE 7.5. High grade mucoepidermoid carcinoma. Papanicolaou stain showing atypical cells with hard squamoid cytoplasm, overlapping nuclei, nuclear pleomorphism, irregular nuclear contours and some prominent nucleoli (400×).

TABLE 7.1. Key diagnostic features of MEC

Variable mixture of the three cell components: mucinous, squamoid, and intermediate cells

Low grade:

- Small clusters of mucinous cells with small round nuclei and abundant vacuolated cytoplasm
- Intermediate cells
- Mucinous background (stains pale purple with Romanowsky stain and pale blue green with Papanicolaou stain)

High grade:

- Large groups and clusters
- Large hyperchromatic nuclei, with irregular nuclear contours and prominent nucleoli
- Numerous cells with squamoid (dense) cytoplasm
- Mucinous cells are rare

Cell blocks can be helpful with the architectural morphology as well as ancillary studies. The architectural morphology will be informative in good quality cell block material and is similar to general histological features. High-molecular-weight cytokeratin immunostain can be used to highlight the squamoid cells, and mucicarmine stain can be used to identify mucinous cells (Table 7.1).

Histologically, low-grade tumors tend to be cystic, well circumscribed, and lined mostly by bland mucinous cells in addition to intermediate and squamoid cells (Figures 7.6 and 7.7). The mucinous cells are large with abundant pale cytoplasm pushing the nucleus to the periphery. The intermediate cells are cuboidal with small, round, centrally placed nuclei. The cytoplasm is pale pink. Scattered squamoid cells with dense eosinophilic cytoplasm are observed. Keratinization and pearl formation is found rarely. Chronic inflammation may be observed around the tumor. High-grade tumors are infiltrative and show solid sheets of intermediate to nonkeratinized squamoid cells with scant mucinous cells (Figure 7.8). Higher degrees of nuclear atypia and an increased mitotic rate and necrosis are noted. Perineural and lymphovascular invasion can be identified readily. Mucicarmine stain can be helpful in identifying the rare mucinous cells to establish the MEC diagnosis.

7.4 DIFFERENTIAL DIAGNOSIS

Low-grade MEC is the most common cause of false-negative diagnosis in salivary gland FNA. Because most low-grade MECs are cystic, adequate

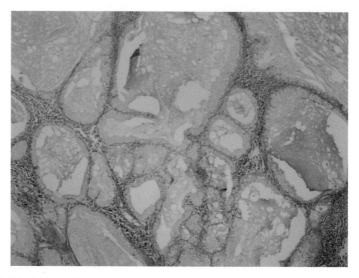

FIGURE 7.6. Low grade mucoepidermoid carcinoma. On H&E the tumor is composed of dilated glandular spaces distended with mucin and lined by bland columnar mucinous cells. Chronic inflammation is noted in the surrounding stroma (100×).

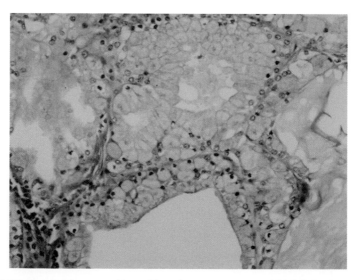

FIGURE 7.7. Low grade mucoepidermoid carcinoma. High power of H&E showing the bland columnar mucinous cells (200×).

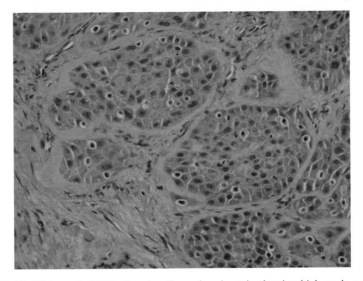

FIGURE 7.8. High-grade MEC. Hematoxylin and eosin stain showing high-grade squamoid cells with well-defined cytoplasmic borders, pleomorphic nuclei, and prominent nucleoli infiltrating the stroma (200×).

sampling is critical to make the correct diagnosis. One of the most important diagnostic considerations is mucous retention cyst or mucocele. A helpful clue in supporting a neoplastic process is the persistence of a mass after aspiration. Usually, MEC is more cellular and the presence of intermediate and squamoid cells is a helpful finding. One also should keep in mind the occurrence of metaplasia in chronic sialadenitis, where both squamous and mucinous metaplasia can be observed. Other tumors that could have mucinous and squamous metaplasia are Warthin's tumor and pleomorphic adenoma. These changes, when present, are usually focal and accompanied by other diagnostic cell components.

Oncocytic cell change can be extensive in MEC and can pose a diagnostic challenge to differentiate them from oncocytic neoplasms of the salivary gland, such as Warthin's tumor, oncocytoma, and oncocytic carcinoma. Again, the squamoid and mucinous component should be identified to diagnose MEC (Table 7.2).

High-grade MEC can mimic other high-grade tumors, such as salivary duct carcinoma, carcinoma ex pleomorphic adenoma, adenosquamous carcinoma, and metastatic squamous cell carcinoma. Identifying glandular and squamous components are required for the diagnosis of MEC. Mucicarmine stain can be helpful to highlight these cells. Carcinoma ex pleomorphic adenoma develops after long-standing history (years) of pleomorphic adenoma, and with proper sampling, the adenoma and carcinoma components might be viewed. Usually, salivary duct carcinoma has extensive necrosis

TABLE 7.2.	
Differential diagnosis of low-grade MEC	Diagnostic clues to make the distinction
Mucous retention cyst (mucocele)	Usually, MEC is more cellular. Look for intermediate and squamoid cells.
Chronic sialadenitis with mucinous metaplasia	Few mucinous cells. Lack of abundant mucin in the background. No intermediate cells. Chronic inflammation, fibrosis and sometimes fragments of stones.
Pleomorphic adenoma with mucinous metaplasia	Few mucinous cells. Other typical features of pleomorphic adenoma (bland epithelial cells intermixed with fibrillary fibromyxoid matrix).
Warthin's tumor with mucinous metaplasia	Few mucinous cells. Watery proteinaceous background not mucinous. Other typical features of Warthin's tumor (oncocytic cells with abundant granular eosinophilic cytoplasm and lymphocytes in the background).

and may show papillary morphology. The presence of extensive keratinization and pearl formation is associated with squamous cell carcinoma rather than MEC. A clinical history of other masses in the head and neck or previous pleomorphic adenoma is helpful. In general, all high-grade primary tumors are treated similarly, so a definitive classification is not that essential (Table 7.3).

7.5 TREATMENT AND PROGNOSIS

Prognosis is related to histological grade, extraglandular extension, necrosis, increased mitosis and presence of metastasis. In one study, low-grade tumors had 97.7% 5-year disease-free survival, whereas high-grade tumors had 28.5% 5-year disease-free survival. The status of resection margins, stage and location are also important prognostic factors. The 5-year cure rate for stages I, II, and III were reported as 97%, 83%, and 28%, respectively. Tumors in the submandibular salivary gland were reported to have more frequent lymph node metastasis, and tumors of the tongue and floor of mouth demonstrated more aggressive behavior. Death results from advanced local disease, distant metastasis, or complications of therapy. Low-grade tumors are treated with wide local excision. High-grade tumors are treated with more aggressive surgery with possible lymph node dissection and radiotherapy. Radiation therapy is indicated for high-grade and high-stage

TABLE 7.3.

Differential diagnosis of high-grade MEC	Diagnostic clues to make the distinction
Salivary duct carcinoma	Look for mucinous component (mucicarmine stain can be helpful). Salivary duct carcinoma usually has extensive necrosis and may show papillary morphology. Cell block may show comedo-type necrosis similar to high-grade ductal carcinoma in situ of the breast.
Carcinoma ex pleomorphic adenoma	Long clinical history of pleomorphic adenoma + admixed pleomorphic adenoma cytological features.
Metastatic squamous cell carcinoma	Look for mucinous component (mucicarmine stain can be helpful). The presence of extensive keratinization and pearl formation is associated with squamous cell carcinoma rather than MEC. Clinical history of other masses in the head and neck.

carcinoma, tumors with extensive perineural and vascular invasion, incompletely excised tumors, and tumors of the deep lobe of parotid gland and base of tongue. The role of chemotherapy is not yet well established.

RECOMMENDED READINGS

Boahene DK, Olsen KD, Lewis JE, Pinheiro AD, et al. Mucoepidermoid carcinoma of the parotid gland: the Mayo Clinic experience. Arch Otolaryngol Head Neck Surg 2004;130:849–856.

Cibas ES, Ducatman BS. Cytology: Diagnostic Principles and Clinical Correlates. Philadelphia (PA): Saunders; 2003.

Daneshbod Y, Daneshbod K, Khademi B. Diagnostic difficulties in the interpretation of fine needle aspirate samples in salivary lesions: diagnostic pitfalls revisited. Acta Cytol 2009;53(1):53–70.

David O, Blaney S, Hearp M. Parotid gland fine-needle aspiration cytology: an approach to differential diagnosis. Diagn Cytopthol 2007;35(1):47–56.

Edwards PC, Wasserman P. Evaluation of cystic salivary gland lesions by fine needle aspiration: an analysis of 21 cases. Acta Cytol 2005;49(5):489–494.

Goonewardene SA, Nasuti JF. Value of mucin detection in distinguishing mucoepidermoid carcinoma from Warthin's tumor on fine needle aspiration. Acta Cytol 2002;46(4):704–708.

Hicks MJ, el-Naggar AK, Flaitz CM, Luna MA, et al. Histocytologic grading of mucoepidermoid carcinoma of major salivary glands in prognosis and survival: a clinicopathologic and flow cytometric investigation. Head Neck 1995;17(2):89–95.

Hughes JH, Volk EE, Wilbur DC. Pitfalls in salivary gland fine-needle aspiration cytology: lessons from the College of American Pathologists Interlaboratory Comparison Program in Nongynecologic Cytology. Arch Pathol Lab Med 2005;129(1):26–31.

Layfield LJ. Fine-needle aspiration in the diagnosis of head and neck lesions: a review and discussion of problems in differential diagnosis. Diagn Cytopthol 2007;35 (12):798–805.

Luna MA. Salivary mucoepidermoid carcinoma: revisited. Adv Anat Pathol 2006;13 (6):293–307.

Mukunyadzi P. Review of fine-needle aspiration cytology of salivary gland neoplasms, with emphasis on differential diagnosis. Am J Clin Pathol 2002;118Suppl: S100–S115.

Rajwanshi A, Gupta K, Gupta N, Shukla R, et al. Fine-needle aspiration cytology of salivary glands: diagnostic pitfalls-revisited. Diagn Cytopthol 2006;34(8):580–584.

Triantafillidou K, Dimitrakopoulos J, Iordanidis F, Koufogiannis D. Mucoepidermoid carcinoma of minor salivary glands: a clinical study of 16 cases and review of the literature. Oral Dis 2006;12(4):364–370.

CHAPTER 8

CARCINOMA EX PLEOMORPHIC ADENOMA

HUSAIN A. SALEH, MD, FIAC, MBA

8.1 INTRODUCTION

Carcinoma ex pleomorphic adenoma is a malignant epithelial tumor of salivary glands arising in preexisting pleomorphic adenoma and accounts for approximately 12% of all malignant salivary gland tumors. It occurs equally in men and women, and it is found mainly in the parotid gland.

8.2 CLINICAL FEATURES

Carcinoma ex pleomorphic adenoma (ca-ex-PA) involves mostly the parotid gland (the most common place of pleomorphic adenoma), followed by minor salivary glands and submandibular gland with equal sex distribution. It comprises approximately 3.6% of all salivary gland tumors, and it is estimated that approximately 10% of PAs become malignant. The patients commonly present in the sixth or seventh decade with a long history of a slowly growing mass in parotid or other site of the neck, and with recent rapid increase in size, pain, or facial paralysis. Sometimes, there is a history of previous surgery or radiotherapy. The malignant transformation might be confined to the gland or might extend beyond the gland to invade surrounding structures.

Occasionally, patients present with a rapidly growing mass without a history of a preexisting mass (de novo ca-ex-PA). This mass has been called by some authors as true malignant mixed tumor or carcinosarcoma, and often it shows ductal carcinoma mixed with chondrosarcoma.

Salivary Gland Cytology: A Color Atlas, Edited by Mousa A. Al-Abbadi
Copyright © 2011 Wiley-Blackwell

8.3   CYTOLOGICAL FEATURES AND HISTOLOGICAL CORRELATION

The aspirate smears of ca-ex-PA usually are cellular and contain dual populations of malignant cells and benign residual PA cells (Figure 8.1). Perhaps because of low cohesion of the tumor cells in the malignant part, the aspirate is dominated usually by malignant cells (Table 8.1). These malignant cells are arranged frequently in loose, irregular clusters or single cells (Figures 8.2 and 8.3). An epithelial component is almost always present and includes discohesive groups or single malignant cells, with glandular or squamous differentiation or undifferentiated cells. Usually, the cells are large and pleomorphic with atypical nuclei featuring an irregular membrane, hyperchromasia, and macronucleoli (Figure 8.4). A malignant stromal cell component may be observed rarely, but it is more difficult to identify than the carcinoma component on cytology aspirates (Figures 8.5 and 8.6). Cell block sections can be helpful in demonstrating microfragments of malignant tumor with both malignant epithelial cells and benign PA cell components (Figure 8.7). A clear presence of benign PA components (uniform small cells and spindle cells in chondromyxoid fibrillary stroma) should be identified microscopically to make this diagnosis, although this is frequently overrun, obscured, or dominated by the malignant component of the tumor.

The tumor ranges from 3 to 12 cm in size and is poorly circumscribed. It may appear encapsulated, but focal areas of capsular disruption and

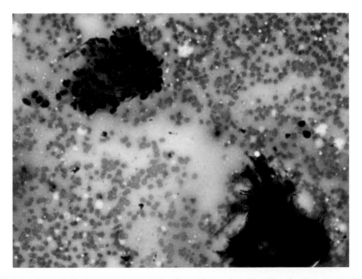

FIGURE 8.1. Ca-ex-PA. Group of atypical cells with overlapping discohesive arrangement and pleomorphic nuclei. An adjacent fragment of fibrillary myxoid stromal tissue of preexisting PA is present (Diff-Quik stain, 400×).

TABLE 8.1. Key Diagnostic Features of Carcinoma Ex Pleomorphic Adenoma

- Aspirate may show abundance of particles with "necrotic" appearance during smearing.
- Cellular aspirate with dual population of benign and malignant cells.
- Usually, the malignant component predominates over benign cytologic component.
- Malignant cells are present in discohesive irregular groups and single cells.
- Malignant epithelial cells have glandular or squamous differentiation or undifferentiated.
- Pleomorphic irregular nuclei with hyperchromasia and prominent nucleoli.
- Rarely, malignant stromal component.
- Neoplastic benign component of PA is identified usually.
- Cellular aspirate showing features of PA with necrosis, hemorrhage, calcification, or mitoses may be a clue of malignant transformation in the tumor.

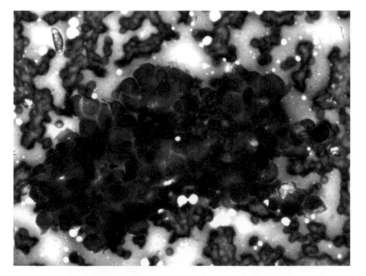

FIGURE 8.2. Ca-ex-PA. A cluster of atypical dispolarized pleomorphic cells with irregular pleomorphic nuclei (Diff-Quik stain, 600×).

infiltration can be found. The cut surface of the tumor resembles PA (firm white tan) but with areas of hemorrhage or necrosis.

Histologically, a ca-ex-PA tumor shows mixed areas of benign PA and areas of poorly differentiated adenocarcinoma or undifferentiated carcinoma in variable proportions (Figure 8.8). However, other types of carcinoma can

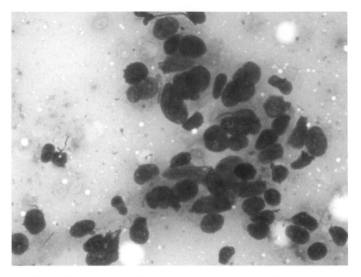

FIGURE 8.3. Ca-ex-PA. A group of discohesive atypical cells with irregular pleomorphic nuclei. The nuclei are overlapping and hyperchromatic (Diff-Quik stain, 600×).

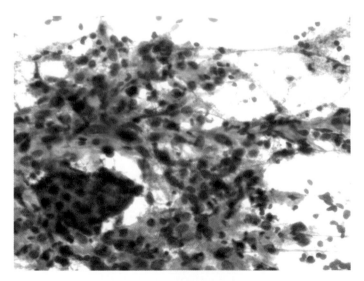

FIGURE 8.4. Ca-ex-PA. A large group of atypical cells in loose three-dimensional arrangement. There is a mixture of apparent epithelial and spindle stromal types of cells with nuclear hyperchromasia and pleomorphism (Papanicolaou stain, 400×).

be identified including salivary duct carcinoma, squamous carcinoma, muco-epidermoid carcinoma, acinic cell carcinoma, or rarely, adenoid cystic carcinoma. Although rare, the stromal component may be malignant (sarcomatous). Occasionally, the benign component is not found, but there is documented history of previously excised PA from the same site. The tumor shows an infiltrative growth pattern with nuclear pleomorphism and hyperchromasia. Usually, tumor necrosis, hemorrhage, and mitoses are identified. Malignancy can be confined to the gland (carcinoma in situ) or can invade through the capsule into surrounding tissue (minimally or widely invasive). The distinction between them is clinically important.

Cytogenetic studies have reported deletions of chromosome 5 and translocation t(10; 12).

8.4 MAJOR CYTOLOGIC DIFFERENTIAL DIAGNOSIS

In general, the cytologic features depend on the histologic subtype of the carcinoma within the mass, and malignant cells usually are observed readily in the aspirate slides. If the benign component is overwhelming in the specimen, then it is recommended to defer final diagnosis to the histologic examination of the resected tumor. When observing a markedly cellular aspirate of PA with evidence of necrosis, hemorrhage, calcification, and mitoses, caution should be taken that a malignancy may be present and should trigger additional thorough tumor sampling and detailed microscopic examination (Table 8.2).

Malignancy should be distinguished from reactive or degenerative changes that can occur in PA. PA with marked cellularity and epithelial atypia is difficult to distinguish from ca-ex-PA. In this situation, surgical resection should be recommended for complete histologic examination and evaluation of stromal or angiolymphatic invasion.

The presence of a stromal component is necessary to distinguish squamous or adenocarcinoma that developed in PA from squamous or adenocarcinoma that developed de novo.

Prior fine needle aspiration (FNA) procedure or spontaneous infarction in an existing PA can result in changes that might be confused with ca-ex-PA. These features include necrosis, hemorrhage, reactive cellular atypia, and background inflammation. The presence of clinical history of prior FNA procedure or occurrence of tenderness because of infarction, as well as a careful review of the cytologic features, including background of infracted tissue, inflammation, and reactive atypia, will help in making the correct cytologic interpretation.

8.5 PROGNOSIS AND TREATMENT

Ca-ex-PA limited to the gland (carcinoma in situ) has excellent prognosis similar to PA. Minimally invasive tumor has good prognosis as well.

TABLE 8.2.

Major cytologic differential diagnoses	Clues to make the distinction
PA with degenerative changes	Lack significant malignant cellular and nuclear features.
	Absence of mitosis, hemorrhage, and necrosis.
	The differential can be difficult and requires focusing on the cellular and nuclear features.
	Surgical resection may be required for final diagnosis.
Spontaneous or post-FNA infarction in PA	Presence of hemorrhage, necrosis, atypical reactive cells and background inflammation (infracted tissue).
	History of previous FNA and local tenderness important.
Salivary duct carcinoma	Poorly differentiated malignant epithelial cells, background necrosis, and mitoses.
	No malignant stromal component.
	No background features of PA.
	No history of preexisting PA.

The widely invasive tumors are aggressive and have poor prognosis with 23% to 50% recurrence rate and up to 70% local or distant metastasis, mostly to lung and bone tissues. The 5-year and 10-year survival rate is 25% to 65% and 18% to 50%, respectively. Tumor size and grade are significant prognostic factors. The estimated 5-year survival rate for undifferentiated carcinoma is 30%, and it is 62% for those with salivary duct carcinoma differentiation.

The treatment of choice is wide local excision with local lymph node dissection. Adjuvant radiotherapy is recommended for widely invasive tumors.

RECOMMENDED READINGS

Al-Khafaji BM, Nestok BR, Katz RL. Fine-needle aspiration of 154 parotid masses with histologic correlation: ten-year experience at the University of Texas M. D. Anderson Cancer Center. Cancer 1998;84(3):153–159.

Daneshbod Y, Daneshbod K, Khademi B. Diagnostic difficulties in the interpretation of fine needle aspirate samples in salivary lesions: diagnostic pitfalls revisited. Acta Cytol 2009;53(1):53–70.

DeMay R. The Art and Science of Cytopathology. Volume II, Aspiration Cytology. Chicago (IL): ASCP Press; 1996. p 676–679.

Ellis GL, Auclair PL. Tumors of the salivary glands. AFIP Atlas of Tumor Pathology, 4th Series, Fascicle 9. Silver Spring (MD): ARP Press; 2008. p 225–246.

Ersöz C, Cetik F, Aydin O, Cosar EF, Talas DU. Salivary duct carcinoma ex pleomorphic adenoma: analysis of the findings in fine-needle aspiration cytology and histology. Diagn Cytopathol 1998;19(3):201–204.

Eveson J. *Malignant neoplasms of the salivary glands.* In: Thompson LD, Goldblum JR, editors. Head and Neck Pathology. Foundation in Diagnostic Pathology. New York: Elsevier; 2006. p 339–345.

Hughes JH, Volk EE, Wilbur DC. Pitfalls in salivary gland fine-needle aspiration cytology: lessons from the College of American Pathologists interlaboratory comparison program in nongynecologic cytology. Arch Pathol Lab Med 2005;129(1):26–31.

Jacobs JC. Low grade mucoepidermoid carcinoma ex pleomorphic adenoma. A diagnostic problem in fine needle aspiration biopsy. Acta Cytol 1994;38(1): 93–97.

Kim T, Yoon GS, Kim O, Gong G. Fine needle aspiration diagnosis of malignant mixed tumor (carcinosarcoma) arising in pleomorphic adenoma of the salivary gland. A case report. Acta Cytol 1998;42(4):1027–1031.

Kwon MY, Gu M. True malignant mixed tumor (carcinosarcoma) of parotid gland with unusual mesenchymal component: a case report and review of the literature. Arch Pathol Lab Med 2001;125(6):812–815.

Nouraei SA, Hope KL, Kelly CG, McLean NR, Soames JV. Carcinoma ex benign pleomorphic adenoma of the parotid gland. Plast Reconstr Surg 2005;116 (5):1206–1213.

Qureshi A, Barakzai A, Sahar NU, Gulzar R, Ahmad Z, Hassan SH. Spectrum of malignancy in mixed tumors of salivary gland: a morphological and immunohis-tochemical review of 23 cases. Indian J Pathol Microbiol 2009;52(2):150–154.

Rajwanshi A, Gupta K, Gupta N, Shukla R, Srinivasan R, Nijhawan R, Vasishta R. Fine-needle aspiration cytology of salivary glands: diagnostic pitfalls — revisited. Diagn Cytopathol 2006;34(8):580–584.

Schindler S, Nayar R, Dutra J, Bedrossian CW. Diagnostic challenges in aspiration cytology of the salivary glands. Semin Diagn Pathol 2001;18(2):124–146.

Stewart CJ, MacKenzie K, McGarry GW, Mowat A. Fine-needle aspiration cytology of salivary gland: a review of 341 cases. Diagn Cytopathol 2000;22 (3):139–146.

CHAPTER 9

ACINIC CELL CARCINOMA

EYAS M. HATTAB, MD and HARVEY M. CRAMER, MD

9.1 INTRODUCTION

According to the 2005 World Health Organization (WHO) classification
of tumors of the salivary glands, acinic cell carcinoma is defined as
"a malignant epithelial neoplasm of salivary glands in which at least some
of the neoplastic cells demonstrate serous acinar cell differentiation, which is
characterized by cytoplasmic zymogen secretory granules. Salivary ductal
cells are also a component of this neoplasm."

Acinic cell carcinoma accounts for approximately 10% of all epithelial
neoplasms of salivary glands, second only to mucoepidermoid carcinoma in
frequency. It is postulated that because the parotid gland is the largest salivary
gland and consists almost exclusively of serous type acini, it is only natural
that it hosts the overwhelming majority of the serous differentiated acinic cell
carcinoma. Previously regarded as "acinic cell tumor," acinic cell carcinoma
is unquestionably malignant.

9.2 CLINICAL FEATURES

Acinic cell carcinoma occurs over a wide age range, affecting children as
young as a few years old and the very elderly with a fairly even age
distribution between the second and seventh decades. Acinic cell carcinoma
is slightly more common in female patients. Most acinic cell carcinomas
involve the parotid gland with a smaller subset of cases occurring in the
intraoral minor salivary glands (buccal mucosa and upper lip). They only are
encountered rarely in the submandibular and sublingual glands. The typical

Salivary Gland Cytology: A Color Atlas, Edited by Mousa A. Al-Abbadi
Copyright © 2011 Wiley-Blackwell

presentation is that of a slowly growing, often painless, unfixed mass in the parotid region with occasional patients manifesting facial nerve palsy. Bilateral examples are rare.

9.3 CYTOLOGICAL FEATURES AND HISTOLOGICAL CORRELATES

9.3.1 Gross Features

Acinic cell carcinomas range from relatively well-circumscribed, solitary nodules to masses that appear ill-defined with irregular edges. Most are about 1–3 cm in the greatest dimension. Their cut surface is tan-red, solid, or cystic and lobulated, with a consistency that varies from soft to firm.

9.3.2 Cytologic Features

The entity, acinic cell carcinoma, derives its name from the presence of numerous disorderly arranged microacinar structures that resemble the normal acini of benign salivary gland tissue (Figure 9.1). Typically, the smear pattern from aspirates of acinic cell carcinoma is loosely cohesive; tightly cohesive epithelial fragments are not seen. Sometimes fibrovascular cores can be identified producing a pseudopapillary appearance. When this occurs, a perivascular growth pattern often is appreciated. Of note, in the usual variety of acinic cell carcinoma, benign ductal epithelial cells are not observed. In most cases, the smear background is clean (Table 9.1).

The tumor cells have abundant cytoplasm and are larger than normal acinar cells. On the Diff-Quik-stained slides, the cytoplasm can be either finely vacuolated or foamy in appearance. However, sometimes the cytoplasm exhibits a granular texture (Figure 9.2). These granules can be either red or basophilic on the Papanicolaou-stained slides (Figure 9.3). Occasionally, the cytoplasm exhibits a dense gray color, conferring an oncocytic appearance to the tumor cells. The cytologic appearance of this tumor closely mirrors the histologic findings (Figure 9.4).

The nuclei, which have a fine to coarse granular chromatin pattern, are round to oval in shape, of medium size, and tend to be centrally located. Occasionally, small nucleoli can be identified. In some cases, numerous naked nuclei may be identified in the smear background. These stripped nuclei reflect the fragile nature of the cytoplasm of the tumor cells and are more likely to be present if harsh smearing techniques are employed. When observed in large numbers, the stripped nuclei may resemble lymphocytes. In other cases, the smear background may contain moderate numbers of true lymphocytes admixed with the neoplastic cells (Table 9.1).

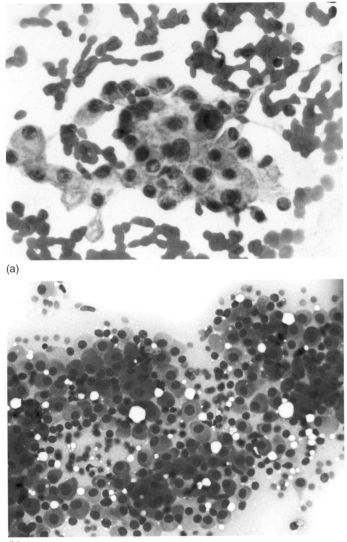

(a)

(b)

FIGURE 9.1. The smear pattern is dominated by characteristic acinar-like architectural arrangements of the tumor cells (**a**, Papanicolaou stain, ×200). In other fields, the tumor exhibits a discohesive smear pattern consisting of numerous large tumor cells with abundant granular cytoplasm and small, round, eccentrically located nuclei (**b**, Diff-Quik stain, ×100).

Despite its subjective nature, grading of acinic cell carcinoma tends to correlate with the tumor's biologic behavior. Higher grade acinic cell carcinomas are characterized by enlargement and irregularity of the nuclei and by an increase in the nuclear:cytoplasmic ratio. Aspirates from moderately differentiated acinic cell carcinomas are more polymorphous

TABLE 9.1. Key diagnostic features of acinic cell carcinoma

Numerous disorderly arranged microacinar structures

Loosely cohesive smear pattern with a clean background

Large cells with abundant, finely vacuolated or foamy cytoplasm

Nuclei are centrally located, round to oval, with fine to coarse granular chromatin

Growth pattern is characterized by sheets or lobules of tumor cells that lack luminal spaces

Nonspecific immunoprofile is reactive for cytokeratins, carcinoembryonic antigen, amylase, and infrequently, S-100 protein

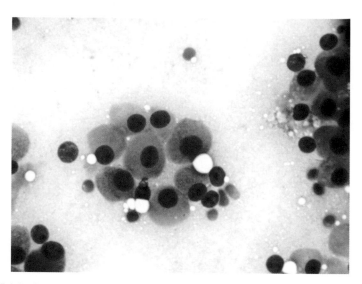

FIGURE 9.2. On medium power, the bland nature of the nuclei and the abundant, fine, granular cytoplasm can be appreciated (Diff-Quik stain, ×200).

in their cytomorphological presentation because they comprise a variety of cell types including duct-like cells, vacuolated cells, and cells with clear cytoplasm. Distinguishing the higher grade acinic cell carcinomas from other high grade salivary gland adenocarcinomas, especially adenocarcinoma not otherwise specified (NOS), can be challenging.

9.3.3 Histopathologic Features

Although acinic cell carcinomas are characterized by serous acinar cell differentiation, several architectural growth patterns and a mixture of

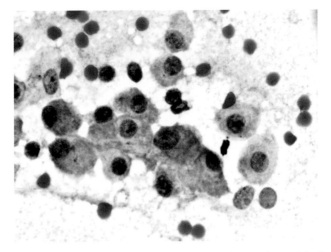

FIGURE 9.3. Numerous small, reddish granules are noted in the cytoplasm of the Papanicolaou-stained slide (Papanicolaou stain, ×400).

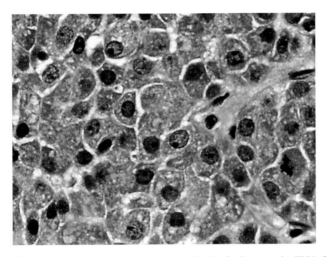

FIGURE 9.4. The histopathologic appearance resembles the findings on the FNA (hematoxylin and eosin stain, ×400).

cell types exist. They may be solid, microcystic, papillary cystic, or follicular. In addition to the acinar cells, cellular constituents include the intercalated ductal, vacuolated, clear, and nonspecific glandular cells. Tumors may show a mixture of these patterns or cell variants or more commonly manifest one pattern and one cell type.

The neoplastic serous acinar cells are large, polygonal with abundant granular pale basophilic cytoplasm, and eccentrically placed, uniform, round nuclei. Similar to normal acinar cells, the cytoplasmic zymogen-like granules are periodic acid Schiff (PAS) positive diastase-resistant, and mucin negative. These stains are especially useful in those tumors in which the acinar cells are a minority. Acinar cell-predominant acinic cell carcinomas are distinguished from normal salivary glands by their sheeting architecture (as opposed to lobular in normal glands), lack of striated ducts, and distended polygonal cytoplasm.

The intercalated duct-like cells are identified in most acinic cell carcinomas but may predominate in up to a third of the tumors. They are somewhat smaller than their acinar counterpart and are typically cuboidal with round, centrally placed nuclei similar in size to those of the acinar cells and often containing a small nucleolus. Unlike the acinar cells, their cytoplasm is eosinophilic to amphophilic. Architecturally, they form back to back, variably sized luminal spaces.

Vacuolated cells may contain one large vacuole that occupies the entire cytoplasm or form multiple small vacuoles with the remaining cytoplasm appearing as eosinophilic to amphophilic. The vacuoles themselves are PAS and mucin negative, although they may contain PAS positive, diastase-resistant, zymogen-like granules. Approximately 10% of acinic cell carcinomas show predominance of vacuolated cells. When identified in salivary gland tumors, vacuolated cells are highly suggestive of acinic cell carcinoma.

Not to be confused with vacuolated cells, clear cells are morphologically similar to acinar neoplastic cells. Clear cells are uncommon in acinic cell carcinoma and only rarely constitute the predominant cell component. Their cytoplasm is PAS negative.

Tumor cells that do not conform to any of the cell types described are termed "nonspecific glandular cells" and are usually polygonal or round with PAS negative, eosinophilic to amphophilic cytoplasm, and round vesicular nuclei. They often form syncytial sheets with ill-defined cytoplasmic borders. They are smaller than the acinar neoplastic cells and on average are more mitotic and pleomorphic.

The solid growth pattern is characterized by sheets or lobules of tumor cells that lack luminal spaces. The serous acinar cells are usually the predominant cell component. The microcystic pattern shows abundance of variably sized cystic spaces that are often clear but occasionally may contain pale proteinaceous material. The solid and microcystic patterns frequently coexist and account for most acinic cell carcinomas. The papillary cystic pattern differs from the microcystic pattern in that the spaces are larger and their lumens contain papillary epithelial proliferations. Depending on the plane of section, the latter may appear "floating" within the cystic spaces. Acinar cells are infrequent in the papillary cystic pattern in which the intercalated duct and vacuolated cells usually predominate. The least common follicular pattern is produced by a thyroid follicle-like proliferation of variably sized, epithelial-lined cystic spaces containing PAS positive, eosinophilic proteinaceous material. This pattern also is dominated by intercalated duct cells.

Psammoma bodies occasionally may be encountered, particularly in the papillary cystic pattern. The stroma of acinic cell carcinoma may be scant or abundantly fibrotic and in many tumors is associated with a prominent lymphoid infiltrate, sometimes forming germinal centers and mimicking nodal tissue. Those tumors that are well-circumscribed and dominated by lymphoid tissue are thought to behave more favorably.

Acinic cell carcinomas do not have a specific immunoprofile. They are reactive for cytokeratins, carcinoembryonic antigen, vasoactive intestinal polypeptide, amylase, and infrequently, S-100 protein.

9.4   CYTOLOGIC DIFFERENTIAL DIAGNOSIS

Because acinic cell carcinoma accounts for as few as 1% of all salivary gland carcinomas, the entity rarely is encountered except in the busiest of head and neck cytology practices. In part, the relative rarity of acinic cell carcinoma contributes to the relatively low fine needle aspiration (FNA) accuracy rates that are reported in the literature.

As a whole, the sensitivity of salivary gland FNA for the diagnosis of salivary gland malignancies is approximately 70%, whereas the specificity of a benign diagnosis is approximately 90%. The accuracy rate for the cytologic diagnosis of acinic cell carcinoma is even less than for other subtypes of salivary gland malignancy. For example, of 22 cases reported by Klija-nienko and Vielh (1997), only three cases were diagnosed definitively as acinic cell carcinoma; 70% of their cases were diagnosed correctly as carcinoma but were subcategorized incorrectly.

According to data obtained from the College of American Pathologists Interlaboratory Comparison Program in Nongynecologic Cytology, the false positive rate for salivary gland FNA is approximately 8%. Pathologists in the United States correctly diagnosed acinic cell carcinomas as being malignant in only 50% cases, and a correct specific diagnosis of acinic cell carcinoma was established by only 40% of participating pathologists. In this survey, almost 50% of the acinic cell carcinoma cases were diagnosed falsely as negative, although it can be argued that the survey used methodologies that varied significantly from standard clinical practice in which access to clinical information and additional cytologic preparations are usually available. The cytologic differential diagnosis of acinic cell carcinoma is relatively extensive, thereby contributing to the relatively frequent sub-classification errors reported in the literature. Careful consideration of the cytomorphological differential diagnosis can reduce the rate of diagnostic errors.

Fine needle aspirates of a normal salivary gland can be a cause of a false positive diagnosis of acinic cell carcinoma, a serious error that can lead to unnecessary surgery and needless patient morbidity. This situation can occur if an unusually vigorous FNA produces an unexpected hypercellular sample. In aspirates from a normal salivary gland, the normal lobular architecture of the acini should be preserved and is admixed with adipose tissue, and some benign ductal elements are often present. Both serous and mucous cells should be observed in aspirates of a normal salivary gland and are not present in acinic cell carcinomas. The acinar-like architectural pattern is the hallmark for the cytologic diagnosis of acinar cell carcinoma, but these acinar-like fragments are larger, less well-defined, more disordered, and less cohesive than those usually observed in aspirates from a normal salivary gland. In acinic cell carcinoma, the neoplastic cellular proliferation is more monomorphic than aspirates of a normal salivary gland.

Sialadenosis is an entity that closely resembles normal salivary gland. This entity is a nonneoplastic enlargement of the salivary glands that is believed to be secondary to secretory dysfunction or other metabolic factors. The main histologic finding is acinar hypertrophy with the accumulation of increased numbers of secretory granules. Aspirates from sialadenosis can be markedly cellular, prompting consideration of acinic cell carcinoma. The cells comprising sialadenosis are larger than those observed in a normal salivary gland, but unlike true acinic cell carcinoma, the normal micro-architectural appearance should be preserved. In false negative aspirates of acinic cell carcinoma, the increased cellularity of the FNA in comparison with a normal salivary gland may not be appreciated, leading to a false impression of a nonneoplastic process.

Fine needle aspirates of acinic cell carcinoma commonly contain cells with clear cytoplasm. The most common salivary gland malignancy, which cytologically can present with numerous clear cells that can be confused with acinic cell carcinoma, is low grade mucoepidermoid carcinoma. The vacuolated cells observed in aspirates from low grade mucoepidermoid carcinoma and acinic cell carcinoma can be indistinguishable from one another. Typically, aspirates from low grade mucoepidermoid carcinoma are more varied in appearance than the monomorphic aspirates of acinic cell carcinoma. They contain a mixture of macrophages, squamous cells, large sheets of so-called intermediate cells, and numerous clear cells. Extracellular mucin is often noted in the smear background of low grade mucoepidermoid carcinoma, whereas mucin is never a feature of aspirates from acinic cell carcinoma. A mucin stain will be positive in low grade mucoepidermoid carcinoma but always will be negative in aspirates from acinic cell carcinoma. Therefore, the absence of extracellular mucin, mucin secreting cells, intermediate cells, or squamous cells would be features in favor of a diagnosis of acinic cell carcinoma for salivary gland aspirates containing large numbers of clear cells. Clear cells also can be observed in aspirates from metastatic renal cell carcinoma, but usually, these patients will present with a prior history of renal cell carcinoma. Epithelial myoepithelial carcinoma also can present with clear cells, but aspirates from these tumors usually present as three-dimensional clusters of basaloid cells with clear cytoplasm in the peripheral cells and acellular hyaline material.

The cells comprising acinar cell carcinomas can be granular, and distinction from oncocytes can be difficult. In oncocytes, the granularity is secondary to the presence of mitochondria, whereas the granules of acinic cell carcinomas are secretory zymogen granules. The granules of oncocytes originating from either a Warthin's tumor or oncocytoma are finer than the granules of acinic cell carcinoma. In acinic cell carcinomas, cells with both vacuolated and nonvacuolated, granular cytoplasm can be observed, whereas true oncocytes are always nonvacuolated. Oncocytes also can show clear cell change, a finding that further complicates cytomorphological interpretation.

In cases in which oncocytoma is considered in the differential diagnosis, performing PAS stain with and without diastase digestion is one method that can be used to distinguish between these two possibilities. In acinic cell carcinoma, diastase-resistant PAS positive granules are identified, whereas oncocytes will not contain any reddish granules after diastase digestion. However, when performing these histochemical stains, it is important to adhere to strict protocol. If there is insufficient diastase digestion, then it may be possible to detect seemingly diastase-resistant PAS positive granules in oncocytoma, thereby leading to a misdiagnosis of acinic cell carcinoma.

Aspirates from acinic cell carcinoma may contain numerous naked nuclei that can be difficult to distinguish from lymphocytes. If the cells comprising the acinic cell carcinoma are mostly granular, then the presence of lymphocyte-like naked nuclei in the smear background could cause confusion with a Warthin's tumor because aspirates from Warthin's tumors characteristically contain groups of oncocytes surrounded by lymphocytes. Furthermore, in some cases of acinic cell carcinoma, a true lymphoid infiltrate may be noted in the smear background, and the presence of true lymphocytes admixed with granular tumor cells also can lead to a misdiagnosis of Warthin's tumor. In most cases, oncocytes have dense, finely granular cytoplasm with well-defined cell borders, findings that are usually but not always distinguishable from the cells of acinic cell carcinoma.

The presence of either naked nuclei or true lymphocytes in the smear background also may prompt a misdiagnosis of chronic sialadenitis, especially if the microacinar architecture that is characteristic of typical acinic cell carcinoma is misinterpreted as true acini of benign salivary gland origin. However, in chronic sialadenitis, the lymphoid infiltrate is usually of modest cellularity.

Acinic cell carcinoma is one of the many salivary gland neoplasms that can undergo cystic change. If the cyst contents are aspirated, then only macrophages may be observed. Often the epithelial component of aspirates from cystic acinic cell carcinomas is hypocellular, making a definitive diagnosis of acinic cell carcinoma very difficult or impossible. All cystic aspirates should be examined carefully for the presence of occasional tubular or spherical aggregates of epithelial cells with vacuolated or granular cytoplasm. If such cells are identified in the presence of a cystic aspirate with numerous macrophages, then the diagnosis of a cystic acinic cell carcinoma can be entertained.

The papillary cystic variant of acinic cell carcinoma can be extremely difficult to diagnose. In a series of seven cases reported by Ali (2002), none were diagnosed correctly by preoperative FNA.

Aspirates from the papillary cystic variant of acinic cell carcinoma are highly cellular and consist of complex architectural patterns. The microacinar pattern that is characteristic for conventional acinic cell carcinoma is not a feature of this variant, and these aspirates do not contain arborizing capillaries or single cells. Instead, the smears contain large, monolayer sheets, sometimes with numerous finger-like papillary projections. In some cases, the cells exhibit an oncocytic appearance that once again can be confused with an oncocytic neoplasm. Because these are cystic neoplasms, the cells within the cyst fluid tend to round up and become vacuolated, and their putative cytomorphological similarity to normal serous acinar epithelium is eliminated. Psammoma bodies may be observed, suggesting the possibility of a metastatic thyroid papillary carcinoma. The cytomorphological differential diagnosis of the papillary cystic variant of acinic cell carcinoma includes mucoepidermoid carcinoma, oncocytoma, Warthin's tumor, cellular pleomorphic adenoma, sebaceous adenoma, and metastatic malignancy.

Grading of fine needle aspirates of acinic cell carcinomas rarely is attempted and, in any case, is a highly subjective exercise. Most aspirates from the usual type of acinic cell carcinomas are low grade. Once the tumor becomes high grade, distinguishing it from other types of salivary gland carcinomas may be very difficult. In fact, most cases of high grade acinic cell carcinoma will be designated by the cytopathologists as adenocarcinoma NOS. Poorly differentiated acinic cell carcinomas are rare and accurately subclassifying them by FNA is problematic. Fortunately, from a clinical standpoint, it is probably not important to distinguish poorly differentiated acinic cell carcinoma from other salivary gland adenocarcinomas because the treatment of higher grade salivary gland carcinomas is the same.

Table 9.2 summarizes the cytological differential diagnosis and the clues to make the distinctions.

9.5   TREATMENT OF CHOICE AND PROGNOSIS

Complete surgical excision is the treatment of choice. The extent of surgical excision is the best predictor of disease-free survival. There is a reported

TABLE 9.2. Cytological differential diagnosis	
	Clues to make the distinction
Oncocytoma	Oncocytes have fine granules and always are nonvacuolated. The absence of PAS granular positivity after diastase digestion differentiates oncocytoma from acinic cell carcinoma which is PAS-D positive.
Warthin's tumor	Warthin's tumor has finer granules than acinic cell carcinoma and contains groups of oncocytes surrounded by lymphocytes.
Low grade mucoepidermoid carcinoma	Low grade mucoepidermoid carcinoma aspirates are more varied in appearance than acinic cell carcinoma, with a mixture of macrophages, squamous cells, large sheets of intermediate cells, and clear cells; mucin stains are positive.
Sialadenosis	Sialadenosis is nonneoplastic and exhibits acinar hypertrophy with an accumulation of increased numbers of secretory granules. Unlike acinic cell carcinoma, the normal microarchitectural appearance is preserved.

incidence of local recurrence of about 35%. Lymph node and distant metastases carry a poor prognosis. There is no consensus on how to grade acinic cell carcinomas, but those tumors with brisk mitotic activity, prominent nuclear pleomorphism, necrosis, infiltration, high proliferative activity, large size, or a deep location seem to behave more aggressively. Tumors developing in minor salivary glands rarely metastasize and as such have a better prognosis than those of major salivary glands. However, acinic cell carcinomas in the submandibular salivary gland are more aggressive than those of the parotid gland.

RECOMMENDED READINGS

Al-Abbadi MA. Letter to the editor. Pitfalls in salivary gland fine-needle aspiration cytology. Arch Pathol Lab Med 2006;130:1428.

Ali SZ. Acinic-cell carcinoma, papillary-cystic variant: a diagnostic dilemma in salivary gland aspiration. Diagn Cytopathol 2002;27:244–250.

Auclair PL, Ellis GL, Stanley MW. Major and minor salivary glands. In: Silverberg SG, Delellis RA, Frable WJ, Virginia AL, Wick MR, editors. Principles and Practice of Surgical Pathology and Cytopathology. 4th ed. New York, NY: Churchill Livingstone; 2006, p 1203–1277.

Cheuk W, Chan JKC. Salivary gland tumors. In: Fletcher CDM, editor. Diagnostic Histopathology of Tumors. 3rd ed. Edinburgh (Scotland): Churchill Livingstone Elsevier; 2007, p 284–288.

DeLellis RA, Frable WJ, LiVolsi VA, Wick MR, editors. Silverberg's Principles and Practice of Surgical Pathology and Cytopathology. 4th ed. Edinburgh (Scotland): Churchill Livingstone/Elsevier; 2006, p 1229–1235.

DeMay RM. Salivary glands. In: DeMay RM, editor. The Art & Science of Cytopathology: Aspiration Cytology. Chicago (IL): ASCP Press; 1996. p 679–680.

Ellis GL, Auclair PL. Malignant epithelial neoplasms: acinic cell adenocarcinoma. In: Ellis GL, Auclair PL, editors. Atlas of Tumor Pathology: Tumors of the Salivary Glands. Washington, DC: Armed Forces Institute of Pathology; 2008, p 204–225.

Ellis G, Simpson RHW. Tumours of the salivary glands. In: Barnes L, Eveson JW, Reichart P, Sidransky D, editors. World Health Organization Classification of Tumours: Pathology and Genetics of Head and Neck Tumours. Lyon (France): IARC Press; 2005, p 216–218.

Hoffman HT, Karnell LH, Robinson RA, Pinkston JA, Menck HR. National Cancer Data Base report on cancer of the head and neck: acinic cell carcinoma. Head Neck 1999;21:297–309.

Hughes JH, Volk EE, Wilbur DC. Pitfalls in salivary gland fine-needle aspiration cytology: lessons from the College of American Pathologists Interlaboratory Comparison Program in Nongynecologic Cytology. Arch Pathol Lab Med 2005;129:26–31.

Klijanienko J. Head and neck; salivary glands. In: Orell SR, Sterrett GF, Whitaker D, editors. Fine Needle Aspiration Cytology. 4th ed. Philadelphia (PA): Elsevier Churchill Livingstone; 2005, p 65–67.

Klijanienko J, Vielh P. Fine-needle sample of salivary gland lesions. V: cytology of 22 cases of acinic cell carcinoma with histologic correlation. Diagn Cytopathol 1997;17:347–352.

Mills SE. Salivary glands. In: Mills SE, Carter D, Greenson JK, Oberman HA, Reuter VE, editors. Sternberg's Diagnostic Surgical Pathology. 5th ed. Philadelphia (PA): Lippincott Williams & Wilkins; 2010, p 839–841.

Mosunjac MB, Siddiqui MT, Tadros T. Acinic cell carcinoma-papillary cystic variant. Pitfalls of fine needle aspiration diagnosis: study of five cases and review of literature. Cytopathology 2009;20:96–102.

Rosai J, Ackerman LV. Epithelial tumors. In: Rosai J, Ackerman LV, editors. Rosai and Ackerman's Surgical Pathology. 9th ed. St. Louis (MO) Mosby; 2004, p 891–892.

Tani EM, Skoog L. Salivary glands and rare head and neck lesions. In: Bibbo M, Wilbur D, editors. Comprehensive Cytopathology. 3rd ed. Philadelphia (PA): Saunders Elsevier; 2008, p 619–621.

Wenig BM. Major and minor salivary glands. In: Wenig BM, editor. Atlas of Head and Neck Pathology. 2nd ed. Philadelphia (PA): Elsevier Saunders; 2008, p 622–628.

CHAPTER 10

BASALOID SALIVARY GLAND TUMOR

JERZY KLIJANIENKO, MD, PHD, MIAC and
ISAM A. ELTOUM, MD, MBA, FIAC

10.1 INTRODUCTION

Basaloid salivary gland tumors are a relatively uncommon group of neoplasms that are morphologically similar but are clinically distinct. They are formed of crowded ovoid cells with a high nuclear cytoplasmic ratio and are devoid of chondromyxoid matrix. They include basal cell adenoma, basal cell adenocarcinoma, solid variant of adenoid cystic carcinoma, cellular pleomorphic adenoma, and other neoplasms.

10.2 BASAL CELL ADENOMA

10.2.1 Introduction

Basal cell adenoma, together with canalicular adenoma, formerly were called "monomorphic adenomas," and are benign salivary tumors. They represent less than 2 % of all salivary neoplasms. Canalicular adenoma is a distinct entity and will not be considered further.

10.2.2 Clinical Features

Basal cell adenoma first was described by Kliensasser and Klein in 1967. It presents commonly in the parotid gland (75%) as a well-circumscribed encapsulated lesion with or without cystic change.

Salivary Gland Cytology: A Color Atlas, Edited by Mousa A. Al-Abbadi
Copyright © 2011 Wiley-Blackwell

10.2.3   Cytological Features and Histological Correlate

The tumor develops from the salivary gland ducts and shows both basal and luminal cell differentiation. Depending on the differentiation and the amount of hyaline matrix, the tumor shows mixture of one of the following histological patterns: (1) trabecular subtype, when solid cords and insular growth of combined luminal and outer basal cells predominate; (2) tubular subtype, when these cords open up with the formation of lumen and slits that may be filled with mucin; (3) solid subtype, when solid nests of basal cells with peripheral palisading predominate; and (4) membranous subtype, when a large amount of hyaline matrix deposits in and around the epithelial nests in the latter (3) variant. The membranous subtype is observed frequently in cases of familial autosomal dominant cylindromas— Brooke-Spiegler syndrome, a syndrome caused by abnormality in CYLD, a tumor suppressor gene located on chromosome 16. The role of this gene remains to be explored in the rest of basal cell and other basaloid tumors. The hyaline matrix is present also in the other subtypes but to a lesser degree. The luminal cells occasionally may show squamoid differentiation, a feature that is often helpful in the diagnostic work-up.

Cytologic diagnosis of basal cell adenoma is challenging and often ends up as descriptive rather than specific. First, it is generally very difficult to differentiate basal cell adenoma from that of basal adenocarcinoma because the latter often presents with bland cytology. Second, it is similarly challenging to differentiate basal neoplasms from solid variants of adenoid cystic carcinoma. In general, the aspirate from basal cell adenoma shows a scant to very cellular smear, and when cystic changes predominate, the specimen may be inadequate The main cytologic features are epithelial cell clusters, rare isolated intact single cells, numerous naked nuclei, and connective tissue fragments. There is an absence of fibrilar chondromyxoid matrix and hyaline cells, cells with abundant plasmacytoid cytoplasm—two features often seen in pleomorphic adenoma. The cell groups are tightly packed and may show peripheral palisading, whorling, luminal formations, and linear arrangements. In large clusters, focal squamous metaplasia with keratinous debris or lumen with mucin may be present. Connective tissue fragments are hyaline or fibrous, without chondromyxoid metaplasia. Red-magenta globules and/or a thick band of hyaline afibrilar material with smooth margins can be demonstrated best with May–Grünwald–Giemsa (MGG) stain (Figures 10.1a–d). This material may surround a large insular nest of predominantly basal cells as in the solid subtype or bound small angulated clusters of cells in the tubulo-trabecular subtype forming a smooth margin. The central part of the epithelial island may show empty spaces with an anastomosing pattern and/or squamous metaplasia (Figure 10.1e–f).

The individual cells are small to intermediate in size. Characteristically, there are two types of cells, a classical basaloid cell and a comparatively larger luminal cell, which has more abundant cytoplasm than the

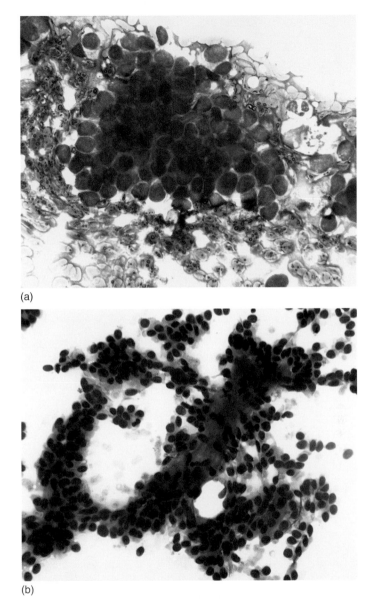

(a)

(b)

FIGURE 10.1. (*Continued*)

former. There is no nuclear atypia, mitosis, or necrosis (Figure 10.1g). Nuclei are rather ovoid than elongated with the shorter diameter on average less than 5.1 μm (less than one red cell diameter). Characteristically, the chromatin is fine and evenly distributed, and the nucleoli are inconspicuous. These nuclear features are particularly prominent in an ultra-fast

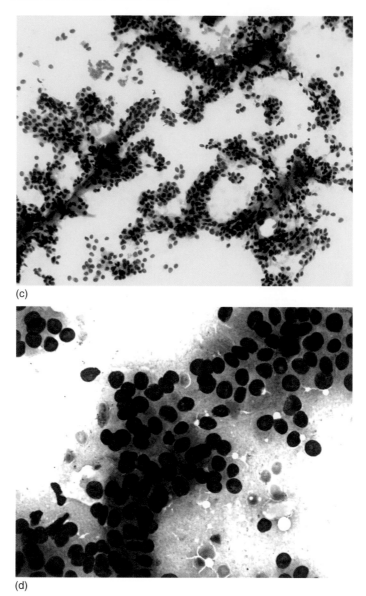

(c)

(d)

FIGURE 10.1. (*Continued*)

Papanicolaou stain, which helps in distinguishing basal cell adenoma from other mimics. Naked nuclei are numerous and identical to nuclei from the epithelial cells. Table 10.1 summarizes the key cellular diagnostic features. The histological sections vary but lack necrosis, frequent mitosis, and significant atypia (Figures 10.1g–i).

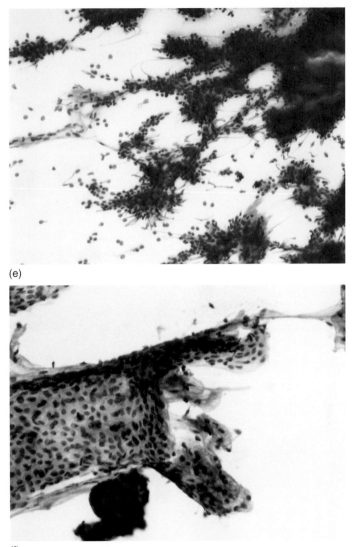

(e)

(f)

FIGURE 10.1. (*Continued*)

10.2.4 Treatment of Choice and Prognosis

Because of its benign behavior, surgical removal with complete free margins is an optimal treatment method. Some basal cell adenomas, especially "membranous subtype," have a tendency to recur. Some investigators believe that it may represent a precursor for carcinoma. However, it is possible that some

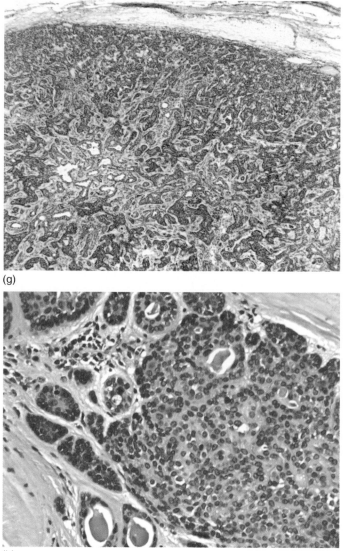

(g)

(h)

FIGURE 10.1. (**a**) Basal cell adenoma: A cluster of uniform basaloid cells with a high nuclear cytoplasmic ratio, scant cytoplasm, and fine chromatin (MGG, 400×). (**b**) Basal cell adenoma: Anastomosing trabeculae formed by uniform cells with bland nuclei. Occasionally, there are cuboidal cells with abundant cytoplasm and polarized nuclei (luminal cells). The nuclear smaller diameter is characteristically smaller than one red blood cell's diameter. Note the connective fragments (MGG, 400×). (**c**) Basal cell adenoma: Large anastomosing trabeculae, connective tissue cords, and background naked nuclei (MGG, 200×). (**d**) Canalicular adenoma. Note the abundant cytoplasm and focal oncocytic metaplasia (MGG, 400×).

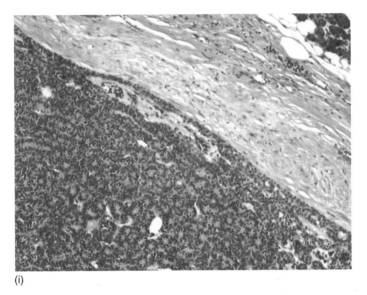

(i)

FIGURE 10.1. (*Continued*) (**e**) Basal cell adenoma: Large anastomosing trabeculae and naked nuclei (Diff-Quik, 200×). (**f**) Basal cell adenoma: Cluster of bland uniform epithelial cells (Papanicolaou stain, 400×). (**g**) Basal cell adenoma: Histological section showing a tubular-trabecular morphology. Note the tumor capsule and the sharp demarcated tumor border (hematoxylin and eosin, 50×). (**h**) Basal cell adenoma: Histological section showing solid and tubular morphology. Note two populations of cells, lumen, and secretions (hematoxylin and eosin, 400×). (**i**) Basal cell adenoma: Histological section showing tubular morphology and capsule formation. Note two populations of cells and lumen (hematoxylin and eosin, 400×).

of these recurring lesions might have been missed cases of solid variants of adenoid cystic carcinoma or might represent the multicentric nature of member-anous basal adenoma especially in the background of Brooke-Spiegler syndrome.

TABLE 10.1. Key diagnostic features of basal cell adenomas
– Basaloid cells with scant cytoplasm
– Nuclear diameter smaller than one red blood cell diameter
– Three-dimensional clusters frequently bounded with a sharp margin hyaline material
– Naked nuclei
– Nonspecific connective tissue fragments
– Bland chromatin
– Squamous cells may be observed
– Hyaline globules

10.3 BASAL CELL ADENOCARCINOMA

10.3.1 Introduction

Basal cell adenocarcinoma is a malignant counterpart of basal cell adenoma. It represents approximately 1% of all salivary neoplasms.

10.3.2 Clinical Features

Basal cell adenocarcinoma occurs in young adults and in older patients. There is no sex predilection, and this tumor occurs exclusively in the major salivary glands.

10.3.3 Cytological Features and Histological Correlate

Basal cell adenocarcinoma is similar to basal cell adenoma and may be divided into solid, trabecular, tubular, and membranous variants. Its distinction as a malignancy is based on the presence of mitotic figures, necrotic areas, and/or the presence of infiltration into the adjacent tissues. Cells are small, round ovoid or elongated with a characteristic peripheral palisading. Nuclei are regular, elongated, and with conspicous nucleoli. The tumor may show squamous metaplasia or hyaline interepithelial deposits. At the periphery, infiltrative growth is observed around branches of the nerves, salivary or muscular tissues, and occasionally in blood vessels.

Cytologically, basal cell adenocarcinomas have characteristic features. Few cases have been reported to date, but all were diagnosed accurately. Tumors consist of three-dimensional clusters of malignant-looking, dark, and round ovoid cells with irregular nuclei and granular chromatin. Glandular and rosette formation are common. Isolated cells are often present. In some cases, mitotic figures are observed. Nuclei often are poorly preserved. Naked nuclei are rare and, when present, are irregular and apoptotic. The hyaline globules frequently are observed within the epithelial clusters. Some cases may show areas of keratin debris or squamous cells (Figures 10.2a–f). The histological correlate demonstrates infiltration, necrosis and frequent mitosis (Figures 10.2g and h).

Basal cell adenocarcinoma should be differentiated from basal cell adenoma and from solid variants of adenoid cystic carcinoma. Difficulties of differential diagnosis are encountered with solid variants of adenoid cystic carcinoma, basal cell adenomas, and basal cell adenocarcinoma when slides contain hyaline globules intimately associated with basaloid clusters. The presence of tubular or finger-like structures, rather than hyaline globules strongly favors adenoid cystic carcinoma. However, in solid variants of adenoid cystic carcinoma, the high mitotic count, coarse chromatin, and comedo-like necrosis readily distinguish

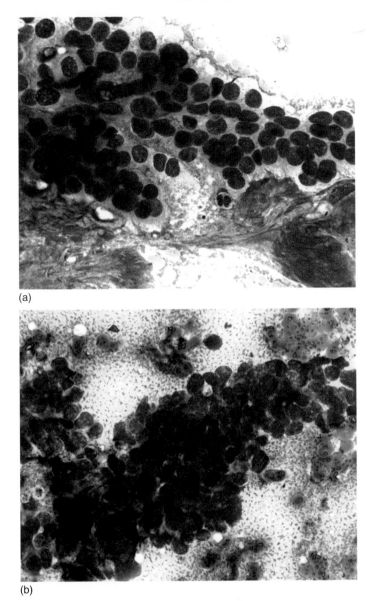

(a)

(b)

FIGURE 10.2. (*Continued*)

adenoid cystic carcinoma from basal cell adenoma and basal cell adenocarcinoma. Hyaline globules may be found in other salivary neoplasms
such as polymorphous low-grade carcinoma, epithelial-myoepithelial
carcinoma, and pleomorphic adenoma. Certain adnexal cutaneous tumors
may contain hyaline globules. Table 10.2 summarizes the key diagnostic
features.

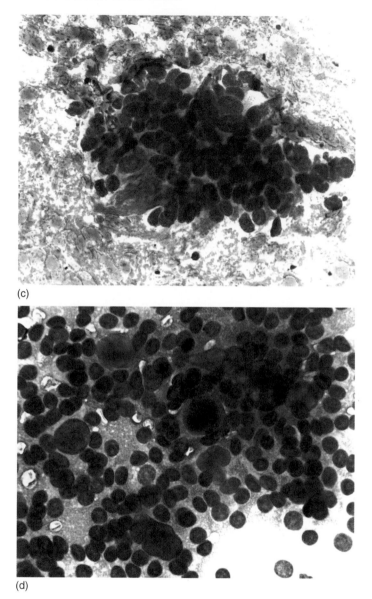

(c)

(d)

FIGURE 10.2. (*Continued*)

10.3.4 Treatment of Choice and Prognosis

A small percentage of tumors metastasize to the lymph nodes. Complete surgical removal is an optimal treatment. The tumor is not likely to respond to radio or chemotherapy.

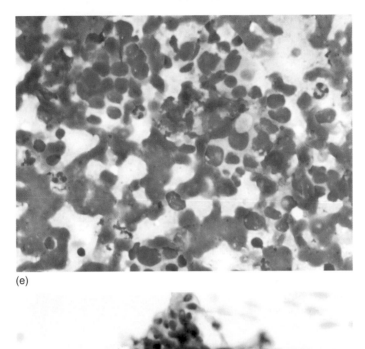

(e)

(f)

FIGURE 10.2. (**a**) Basal cell adenocarcinoma: Note similarity to basal cell adenoma. The cells are slightly larger and vary in their shape. The chromatin is also a little coarse (MGG, 400×). (**b**) Basal cell adenocarcinoma: Nuclear crowding, molding, smudging, and fragmentation. The malignant and seminecrotic feature of these cells is evident (MGG, 400×). (**c**) Basal cell adenocarcinoma: similar to 2B with necrotic nuclear fragments. Note the variation of nuclear size, coarse chromatin, and connective tissue fragments (MGG, 400×). (**d**) Basal cell adeno- carcinoma: Hyaline globules simulating adenoid cystic carcinoma. Note the bland nature of nuclei (MGG, 400×). (**e**) Basal cell adenocarcinoma: Nuclear enlargement, size variations, and fragmentation. Also note the glandular differentiation (MGG, 400×). (**f**) Basal cell adenocarci- noma: Clusters of highly atypical cells with nuclear enlargement, variation nuclear size, and prominent nucleoli compared with a nearby normal acinus (Papanicolaou stain, 400×).

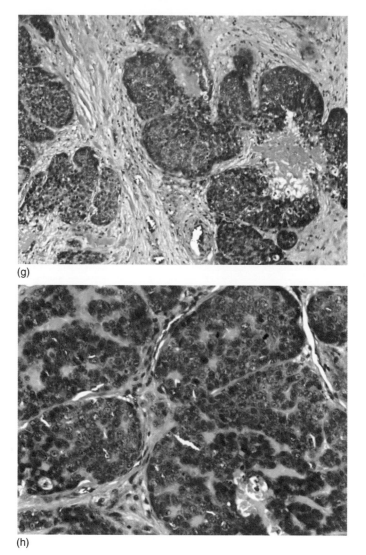

(g)

(h)

FIGURE 10.2. (*Continued*) (**g**) Basal cell adenocarcinoma: Histological section of a solid variant of basal cell adenocarcinoma. Note peripheral pallisading (hematoxylin and eosin, 200×). (**h**) Basal cell adenocarcinoma: Histological section of a solid variant of basal cell adenocarcinoma, high nuclear grade, and mitosis (hematoxylin and eosin, 400X).

10.4   SOLID VARIANT OF ADENOID CYSTIC CARCINOMA

10.4.1   Introduction

In poorly differentiated variants, especially when a solid pattern predominates, adenoid cystic carcinoma becomes difficult to diagnose. Unlike basal

TABLE 10.2. Key diagnostic features of basal cell adenocarcinoma
– Basaloid clusters of dark cells with cellular and nuclear pleomorphism
– Mitoses
– Necrosis
– Naked nuclei
– Squamous cells may be observed
– Hyaline globules

cell adenoma or basal cell adenocarcinoma, adenoid cystic carcinoma with focal solid areas is more frequently encountered in practice. However, pure solid variants are very rare. Depending on the predominance of one of three histological features, adenoid cystic carcinoma is divided into three variants — cribriform, tubular, or solid variants.

10.4.2   Clinical Features

Similar to the basaloid tumors, it occurs most often in both major and accessory salivary glands of elderly patients. The tumor is highly invasive and unpredictable. It grows diffusely and infiltrates the perineural space and the adjacent bones. In advanced cases, it metastasises more frequently to the lung than to lymph nodes.

10.4.3   Cytological Features and Histological Correlate

Solid (poorly differentiated) areas of adenoid cystic carcinoma are morphologically distinct; cells are isomorphic, small, more or less round, and dark. They are arranged in nests and sheets that may show central comedo-like necrosis. In the better differentiated areas, hyaline globules are present. Squamous metaplasia is absent and mitotic figures are frequent.

On cytologic examination, a solid variant of adenoid cystic carcinoma shows cellular smears containing epithelial cell groups and stromal fragments. Cells are arranged in solid sheets and tubular- and finger-like structures. The individual cells are round and dark with a high nuclear cytoplasmic ratio. Nuclei are irregular with small nucleoli. The chromatin is usually coarse. Mitotic figures are frequent. Cells may have scant blue cytoplasm. Naked and sometimes necrotic nuclei may present. In the background, hyaline intensely red-stained globules could be demonstrated on MGG stain (Figures 10.3a–e). The histological correlate shows solid areas of bland basaloid cells (Figure 3f).

10.4.4 The Major Cytological Differential Diagnosis and How to Resolve It

Basal cell adenocarcinoma and pleomorphic adenoma, in its cellular variant, *simulates* solid variants of adenoid cystic carcinoma. The presence of a chondromyxoid background and esspecially the presence of plasmacytoid

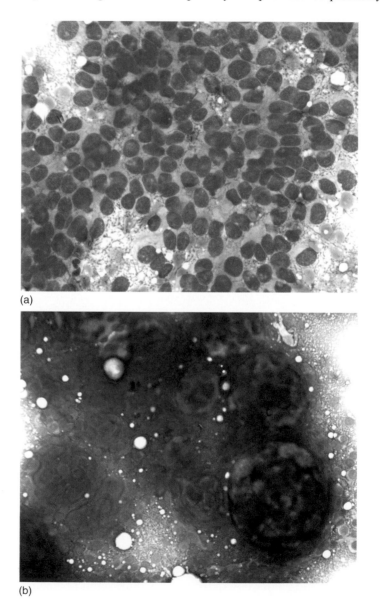

(a)

(b)

FIGURE 10.3. (*Continued*)

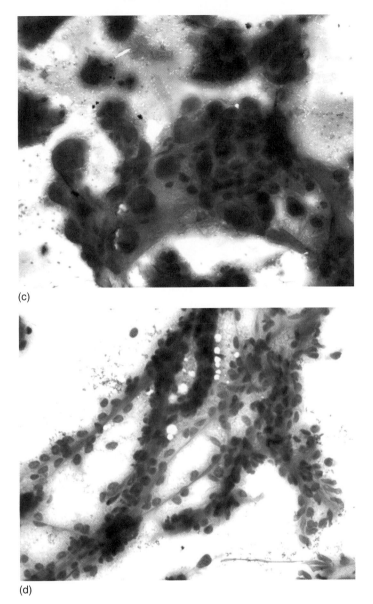

(c)

(d)

FIGURE 10.3. (*Continued*)

myoepithelial cells with abundant cytoplasm favor the diagnosis of pleomorphic adenoma. Metastases of basaloid squamous cell carcinoma (Figures
13.6 and 27), undifferentiated carcinoma of nasopharyngeal type and metastases from thyroid well-differentiated follicular carcinoma, can be mistaken
for solid variant adenoid cystic carcinoma; in these circumstances, the clinical

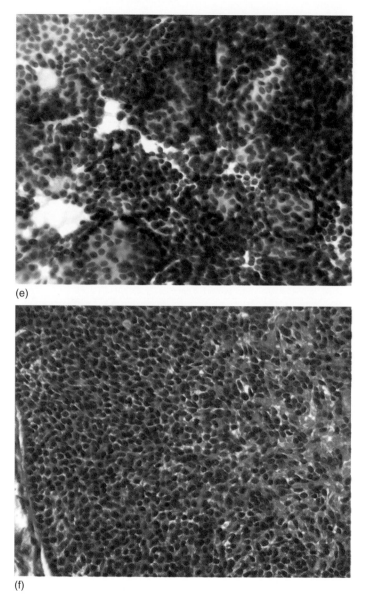

(e)

(f)

FIGURE 10.3. (**a**) A solid variant of adenoid cystic carcinoma—basaloid cells. Note the similarity to basal cell adenocarcinoma (MGG, 400×). (**b**) A solid variant of adenoid cystic carcinoma with characteristic hyaline globules (MGG, 200×). (**c**) A solid variant of adenoid cystic carcinoma. Note the hyaline globule and cribriform pattern (MGG, 100×). (**d**) A solid variant of adenoid cystic carcinoma. The tubular structures are characteristic for adenoid cystic carcinoma (MGG, 400×). (**e**) A solid variant of adenoid cystic carcinoma with solid areas in adenoid cystic carcinoma (hematoxylin and eosin, 200×).

TABLE 10.3. Key diagnostic features of solid variant of adenoid cystic carcinoma

- Basaloid cells in three-dimensional clusters
- Hyaline globules and tubular- and finger-like structures
- Naked nuclei
- Mitoses and cellular and nuclear atypia
- Necrosis

---

information will be most helpful. Table 10.3 summarizes the key cellular diagnostic features.

10.4.5   Treatment of Choice and Prognosis

Complete surgical removal is the optimal treatment. Surgery for adenoid cystic carcinoma is usually more extensive than that required for basal cell adenocarcinoma, which is a reason why the distinction between these entities is important. This tumor is poorly sensitive to radio or chemotherapy.

10.5   POORLY DIFFERENTIATED NEUROENDOCRINE TUMOR (SMALL CELL CARCINOMA)

10.5.1   Introduction

Poorly differentiated neuroendocrine (small cell) carcinoma is a variant of a larger group of salivary carcinomas named "undifferentiated carcinoma." It has identical morphology to its pulmonary counterpart. This entity is rare and represents less than 10% of all salivary carcinomas. In addition, primary small cell carcinoma of salivary glands has to be diagnosed after the exclusion of similar malignancies elsewhere.

10.5.2   Clinical Features

Usually patients present with a large, painful, and fixed parotid mass with regional lymph nodes involvement.

10.5.3   Cytological Features and Histological Correlate

Cytologically, poorly differentiated neuroendocrine (small cell) carcinoma shows characteristic features on smears. The smears are cellular with abundant necrosis and smearing artifacts. Rosette formations and nuclear molding suggest its neuroendocrine origin (Figure 10.4). The cytoplasm is scant and nucleoli are inconspicuous. Histologically, this tumor is identical to pulmonary small cell carcinoma. Cells are medium to large in size with atypical nuclei and an absence of nucleoli. The chromatin is coarse and mitotic figures are common. Table 10.4 summarizes the key cellular diagnostic features.

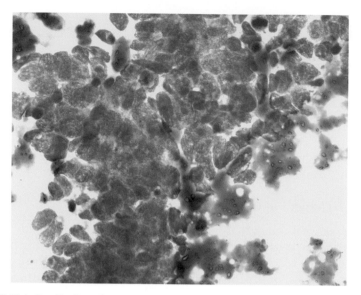

FIGURE 10.4. Small cell carcinoma comprising necrotic and highly malignant cells. Nuclei are inconspicuous (MGG×400).

TABLE 10.4. Key diagnostic features of poorly differentiated neuroendocrine (small cell) carcinoma
– Little or no cytoplasm
– Immature nuclei with inconspicuous nucleoli
– Nuclear molding
– Focal or extensive necrosis
– Mitotic figures
– Rosette-like formations

10.5.4   Treatment of Choice and Prognosis

These tumors are treated aggressively by surgery, chemotherapy, and radiotherapy.

10.6   OTHER POSSIBLE, MUCH LESS COMMON DIFFERENTIAL DIAGNOSES OF BASALOID TUMORS

Other tumors that may mimic these lesions include basaloid tumors of the skin and skin appendages that may present deep in the skin overlying the salivary glands. Smears from basal cell carcinoma of the skin show large anastomosing sheets of tightly cohesive dark epithelial cells with a high nuclear cytoplasmic ratio (Figures 10.5a and b). Occasionally, the cytoplasm may be abundant with focal squamoid differentiation. Single cells are sparse or absent. Mitotic and apoptotic figures are present. Sweat glands and hair follicle tumors may be difficult to differentiate based on cytology alone. Clinical history and physical examination helps in reaching the appropriate diagnosis.

Sialobalstoma is another basaloid tumor that is present exclusively in young children. It is an aggressive lesion with cytologic features that are

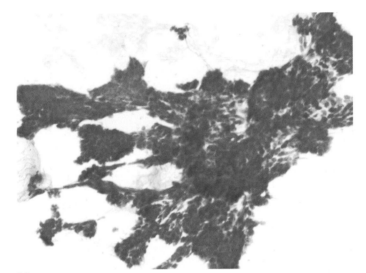

(a)

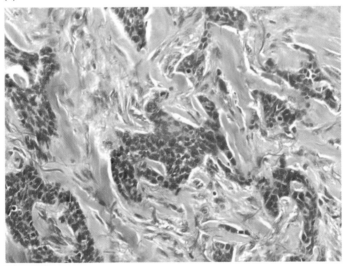

(b)

FIGURE 10.5. (*Continued*)

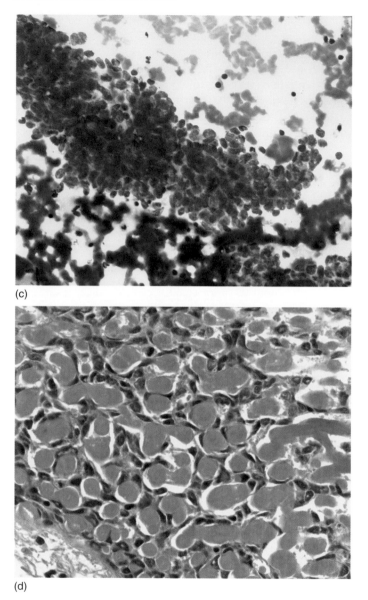

(c)

(d)

FIGURE 10.5. (**a**) Invasive basal cell carcinoma of the skin overlaying the parotid with a deep invasion. Note the anastomosing bands of large basal cells with focally abundant cytoplasm and with irregular and necrotic basaloid cells (Diff-Quik, 200×). (**b**) Basal cell carcinoma of the skin invading the parotid gland (hematoxylin and eosin, 400×). (**c**) Metastatic basaloid squamous cell carcinoma with irregular and necrotic basaloid cells (MGG, 200×). (**d**) Metastatic basaloid squamous cell carcinoma and the corresponding histology (hematoxylin and eosin, 400×).

similar to basal cell adenocarcinoma formed by cell clusters in various arrangements, hyaline globules, two populations of cells, and numerous single cells. Acinar and ductal differentiation may be present.

Finally, metastases of basaloid squamous cell carcinoma (Figure 5.3 to 4), an undifferentiated carcinoma of nasopharyngeal type, and thyroid well-differentiated follicular carcinoma are other entities to be differentiated based on clinical information

In conclusion, basaloid tumors are challenging and may be difficult to diagnose. Table 10.5 summarizes the main differential diagnoses of basaloid tumors of salivary glands and the salient cytological features that help in reaching the correct diagnosis.

TABLE 10.5. Major differential diagnoses of basaloid salivary gland tumors

	Diagnostic clues to make the distinction
Basal cell adenomas	Necrosis and mitotic figures are absent. Numerous naked nuclei and nonspecific connective tissue fragments may help in the differential diagnosis. Canalicular adenoma, however, occurs mainly in the upper lip.
Basal cell adenocarcinoma	Basal cell adenocarcinoma do not show tubular- and finger-like structures, and most exhibit necrosis and nucleoli
Pleomorphic adenoma	The presence of plasmacytoid-like cells with abundant cytoplasm and eccentric nuclei in association with a chondromyxoid matrix strongly favors pleomorphic adenoma.
Solid variant of adenoid cystic carcinoma	Numerous clusters of irregular, dark cells with cellular and nuclear atypia. Mitoses and hyaline globules with tubular- and finger-like patterns.
Metastatic small cell carcinoma	Significant cellular and nuclear pleomorphism with nuclear molding and chromatin smearing. Frequent mitosis. Clinical data will help. Primary versus metastatic is indistinguishable.
Basal cell carcinoma (skin)	Tight clusters, spindle cells, and palisading. History and physical examination are critical.
Sialoblastoma	Young child or infant. Similar to basal cell carcinoma. Acinar and ductal differentiation may be present.
Skin appendage tumors	Syringoma, trichoblastoma, or trichoepithelioma. History, physical examination, and sensitive imaging will have clues.

RECOMMENDED READINGS

Bignell GR, Warren W, Seal S, Takahashi M, Rapley E, Barfoot R, Green H, Brown C, Biggs PJ, Lakhani SR, et al. Identification of the familial cylindromatosis tumour-suppressor gene. Nat Genet 2000;25:160–5.

Dadrick I. Color Atlas/Text of Salivary Galnd Tumor Pathology. New York: Igaku-Shoin Medical Publishers; 1996.

Hara H, Oyama T, Saku T. Fine needle aspiration cytology of basal cell adenoma of the salivary gland. Acta Cytol 2007;51:685–691.

Huang R, Jaffer S. Imprint cytology of metastatic sialoblastoma. A case report. Acta Cytol 2003;47:1123–6.

Kleinsasser O, Klein HJ. Basal cell adenoma of the salivary glands. Arch Klin Exp Ohren Nasen Kehlkopfheilkd 1967;189:302–316.

Klijanienko J, Lagacé R, Servois V, Lussier C, El-Naggar AK, Vielh P. Fine-needle sampling of primary neuroendocrine carcinomas of salivary glands: cytohistological correlations and clinical analysis. Diagn Cytopathol 2001;24:163–6.

Klijanienko J, Vielh P. Fine-needle sampling of salivary gland lesions. III. Cytologic and histologic correlation of 75 cases of adenoid cystic carcinoma: review and experience at the Institut Curie with emphasis on cytologic pitfalls. Diagn Cytopathol 1997;17:36–41.

Klijanienko J, Vielh P, Batsakis JD, el-Naggar AK, Jelen M, Piekarski JD. Salivary gland tumours. Monogr Clin Cytol 2000;15:III–XII, 1–138.

Klijanienko J, Warren W, Seal S, Takahashi M, Rapley E, Barfoot R, Green H, Brown C, Biggs PJ, Lakhani SR, et al. Detection and quantitation by fluorescence in situ hybridization (FISH) and image analysis of HER-2/neu gene amplification in breast cancer fine-needle samples. Cancer 1999;87:312–318.

Yang GC, Waisman J. Distinguishing adenoid cystic carcinoma from cylindromatous adenomas in salivary fine-needle aspirates: the cytologic clues and their ultrastructural basis. Diagn Cytopathol 2006;34:284–8.

CHAPTER 11

ADENOID CYSTIC CARCINOMA

HUSAIN A. SALEH, MD, FIAC, MBA

11.1 INTRODUCTION

Adenoid cystic carcinoma (ACC) is a rare, slow-growing, but relentless malignant neoplasm comprising 3–5% of all salivary gland tumors. It is the most common primary malignancy of all salivary glands except the parotid. It is made up of small bland cells (basaloid epithelial cells and myoepithelial cells) forming variable growth patterns, most commonly a classic cribriform pattern containing hyaline globules. Growth along and invasion of nerves is characteristic.

11.2 CLINICAL FEATURES

ACC occurs mostly in adults in the fourth and fifth decades, although it can occur at any age. It is more common in women than in men with a ratio of approximately 3:2. There has been considerable variability of its incidence among various studies and in different geographic areas. According to the Armed Forces Institute of Pathology (AFIP) and other reports, its incidence is exceeded only by that of mucoepidermoid carcinoma. Its relative incidence is 10% of all salivary gland carcinomas and probably has decreased slightly in recent years because of the emergence of new entities and because of reclassification of salivary gland tumors. It accounts for approximately 4.4% of all major salivary glands tumors and only 1.2% of all parotid tumors. About 25% of ACC involve the major salivary glands (in particular, the submandibular gland), and 75% involve minor salivary glands (especially those in the palate). Interestingly, this tumor also is known to involve other organs such as the trachea, breast, lung, lacrimal and sweat glands, and others.

Salivary Gland Cytology: A Color Atlas, Edited by Mousa A. Al-Abbadi
Copyright © 2011 Wiley-Blackwell

Clinically, more than half of the patients initially present with an asymptomatic painless firm mass that is indistinguishable from other benign or malignant salivary gland tumors. Later, the tumor usually causes tenderness, pain, and facial nerve paralysis. The pain and paralysis from perineural invasion actually may help in making an early diagnosis. The tumor seems fixed to underlying tissue because of marked tumor infiltration in the skin, mucosa, and surrounding structures. Those involving the oral cavity commonly show mucosal ulceration over the mass. Despite its slow growth, it has a poor prognosis because of its relentless long-term growth and difficulty of complete surgical resection resulting from wide infiltration around nerves and surrounding structures. ACC is known to have late metastasis to the lung and bone, and it frequently involves adjacent lymph nodes by direct extension rather than true metastasis. True metastasis to distant lymph nodes is rare.

11.3 CYTOLOGIC FEATURES AND HISTOLOGIC CORRELATION

Typically, the aspirated material in ACC has a mucoid or glistening appearance that may be similar to that of pleomorphic adenoma (PA). The aspirate is usually moderately cellular and shows unique cytologic features with glands, microcysts, cords, and well-outlined solid clusters, and a few singly dispersed cells. The cells are small and deceptively banal appearing. Mitoses are rare. The most characteristic feature is clusters of small, uniform round–oval cells surrounding central cores of homogenous material resembling cribriform structures (Figures 11.1 and 11.2). The homogenous globules may be obscured

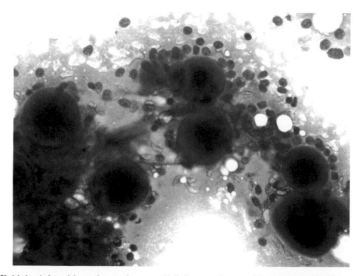

FIGURE 11.1. Adenoid cystic carcinoma. Cellular specimen with clusters of cells containing a round acellular hyaline material that stains metachromatic magenta (Diff-Quik, ×100).

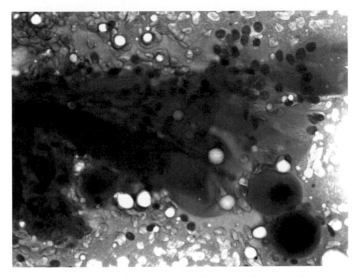

FIGURE 11.2. Adenoid cystic carcinoma. A large cluster of cells surrounding a metachromatic hyaline globule. The cells are uniform bland with round–oval nuclei (Diff-Quik, ×600).

by the thick cell clusters and require adjusting the microscopic focus. The quantitative relationship of the epithelial component and the acellular material varies widely between tumors. Sometimes, cords of the mucoid haylinized material have adherent rows of uniform small cells, a feature that is unique to adenoid cystic carcinoma and helps distinguish this tumor from other primary salivary gland tumors.

The epithelial cells appear as tightly packed, basaloid, small, round to oval, and uniform. The cytoplasm is scant pale, and the nuclear/cytoplasmic (N/C) ratio is high. Their nuclei are small, round–oval, bland, and hyperchromatic with a smooth membrane and small conspicuous nucleoli.

The myoepithelial cells produce the mucoid substance, which stains metachromatic magenta on Diff-Quik stain and stains pale translucent on hematoxylin and eosin or Papanicolaou stains. This substance is similar to the myxoid material observed on smears of PA that also is produced by myoepithelial cells. However, although the substance is homogenous, glassy, or hyaline in ACC, it appears as myxofibrillary and irregular in PA (Figures 11.3 and 11.4).

Hyaline globules are the most characteristic feature of ACC. They appear as round casts, balls, or cylinders of acellular homogenous mucoid material or as branching fronds and columns with rounded contours. They may be surrounded by a layer of small cells (Table 11.1). Cell block sections can be very helpful in showing microfragments with the classic cribriform pattern (Figure 11.5). Rarely, fine needle aspiration biopsy (FNAB) of ACC may lack hyaline globules (as in the solid variant). In general, in aspirates of ACC, as the

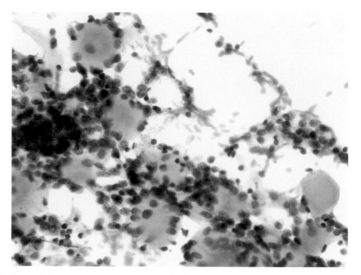

FIGURE 11.3. Adenoid cystic carcinoma. Cellular aspirate with clusters of uniform cells containing and surrounding amorphous hyaline globules (Papanicolaou, ×400).

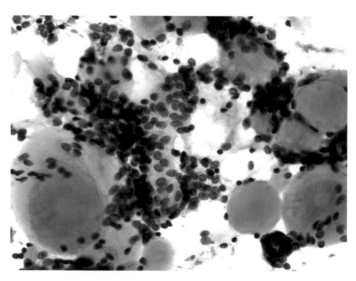

FIGURE 11.4. Adenoid cystic carcinoma. Higher magnification shows groups of uniform cells with an adherent pale amorphous material (hyaline globules). The nuclei are round–oval angulated with a fine chromatin pattern (Papanicolaou, ×600).

amount of hyaline globules decreases, the cellularity, single cells, and cytologic atypia increases. When hyaline globules are scant or absent, the differential with PA and monomorphic adenoma (basal cell adenoma) becomes very important and difficult to assess. However, hyaline globules are not necessary

TABLE 11.1. Cytologic features of adenoid cystic carcinoma

- The aspirate has a thick mucoid appearance
- Cellular aspirate. Glands/microcysts and cords or nests. Few single cells
- Cells are small, basaloid, and deceptively bland.
- Rare mitoses
- Clusters of uniform cells surrounding amorphous hyalinized globules
- Epithelial cells: small and uniform with scant pale cytoplasm and a high N/C ratio. Round–oval hyperchromatic nuclei
- Myoepithelial cells: produce and surround homogenous hyaline globules
- IHC: Dual cell populations. Pankeratin, CK7 and CK19, CEA and EMA stain ductal epithelial cells. Basal cytokeratins such as CK5 and CK17, vimentin, muscle-specific actin, myosin, p63, smooth muscle actin, and calponin stain Myoepthelial cells

or sufficient for the diagnosis and are not specific of ACC. They can be observed in any tumor containing myoepithelial cells including mucin-producing adenocarcinoma, acinic cell carcinoma, PA, myoepithelioma, trabecular adenoma, intraductal papilloma, polymorphous low-grade carcinoma, and epithelial-myoepithelial carcinoma.

ACC have a spectrum of histomorphology and, therefore, can have variable cytomorphologic pictures on FNAB. In addition to the classic appearance already mentioned (small bland cells with hyaline globules), the

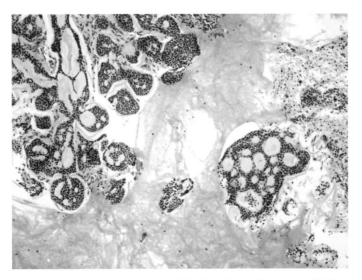

FIGURE 11.5. Adenoid cystic carcinoma. Cell block section with a classic cribriform structure having round microcysts filled with hyaline globules. The cells are uniform and relatively bland (hematoxylin and eosin, ×100).

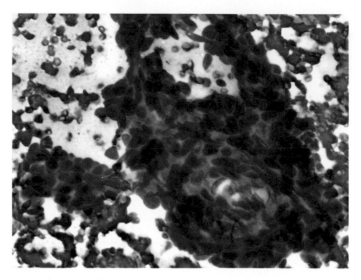

FIGURE 11.6. Adenoid cystic carcinoma, a solid variant. three-dimensional discohesive clusters of cells with no clear hyaline globules. The nuclei show more variation, irregularity, and hyperchromasia than in the ACC cribriform variant (Diff-Quik, ×400).

FNAB of the solid variant will reveal discohesive groups of atypical cells with irregular nuclei and many singly dispersed cells. Hyaline globules are absent or scarce (Figures 11.6 and 11.7). Accurate classification of this clearly malignant tumor on FNAB will be difficult, and the differential will include tumors such as small cell carcinoma, poorly differentiated carcinoma, basal cell adenocarcinoma, basal cell carcinoma, and lymphoma.

In recent years, the liquid-based monolayer cytologic preparation method has been used increasingly in nongynecologic cytology samples including FNAB of salivary glands. Several published studies compared the cytologic features of salivary gland tumors by this method and found certain differences compared with that of the traditional smears. In general, the diagnostic accuracy of this method also has been reported to be similar or higher than that of traditional smears.

Grossly, the tumor is typically circumscribed unencapsulated and forms a firm infiltrative mass. Despite its name, this tumor is only rarely grossly cystic, and the cut surface is white or tan and firm. Histologically, the tumor is polymorphous and has variable growth configurations, but more often, a mixture of growth patterns is common in a single tumor. The type of growth pattern is believed to impact the tumor behavior and prognosis. The classic pattern is *cribriform* resembling "Swiss cheese" and is made up of bland small basoloid epithelial cell and the much more numerous myoepithelial cells (Figure 11.8). The small circular or pseudocyst spaces

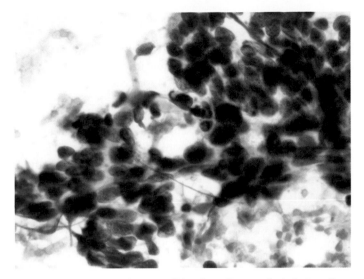

FIGURE 11.7. Adenoid cystic carcinoma, solid variant. Groups of relatively uniform cells with no associated hyaline globules. The nuclei are overlapping, more irregular, hyperchromatic, and angulated than in the cribriform variant (Papanicolaou, ×600).

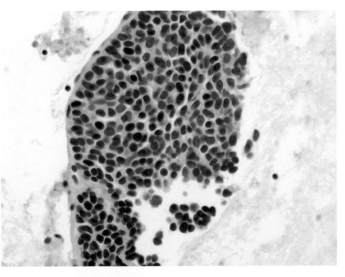

FIGURE 11.8. Adenoid cystic carcinoma, solid variant. Cell block section of a solid variant of adenoid cystic carcinoma with a cohesive three-dimentional group of basaloid cells with a rounded border. Notice the round–oval hyperchromatic nuclei with occasional nucleoli (hematoxylin and eosin ×200).

contain basophilic amorphous material, eosinophilic hyalinized basal lamina material, or both (hence, the name adenoid microcystic carcinoma). The basophilic material stains positively with Alcian blue, whereas the eosinophilic basement membrane-like substance is periodic acid Schiff (PAS) positive. A typical perineural invasion may extend beyond the tumor mass and cause frequent recurrences. Although the latter feature is not specific to ACC, the diagnosis is usually doubtful if it is absent. In addition, there are scattered and small true glands lined by bland ductal epithelial cells, but these glands are few and easily overlooked. The myoepithelial cells have indistinct cytoplasm and round-to-angular nuclei with a homogenous or basophilic chromatin pattern.

Other growth patterns include tubular and solid. The tubular pattern shows more lumens or glands lined by ductal epithelial cells. The characteristic angular nuclei and clear cytoplasm are observed easily. When the eosinophilic hyalinized material is so abundant, it may compresses on the cells forming a trabecular growth pattern.

The solid variant is the least common but is considered the most aggressive form. It shows solid nests or lobules and scant pseudocysts or spaces. The cells are somewhat larger with larger nuclei and frequent mitoses. Tumor necrosis and cellular pleomorphism is often present and indicates a poor prognosis. Focal cribriform or tubular patterns usually are observed (Figure 11.9). This variant can be difficult to distinguish from other basaloid tumors in the head and neck region. Immunohistochemical (IHC) stains will

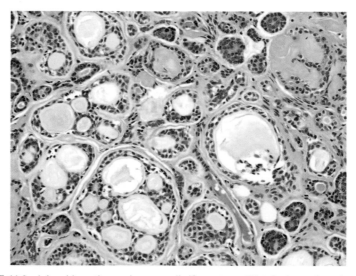

FIGURE 11.9. Adenoid cystic carcinoma, cribriform type. Histologic section showing the classic round pseudocysts filled with pale mucoid or eosinophilic basal-like material. The cells are monotonous and the stroma is hyalinized (hematoxylin and eosin, ×100).

show a dual population of cells in this tumor. pankeratin, cytokeratin 7, and cytokeratin 19 stain the ductal epithelial cells much more intensely than the myoepithelial cells. Carcinoembryonic antigen (CEA) and epithelial membrane antigen (EMA) stain the ductal luminal cells. Myoepthelial cells react positively with basal cytokeratins such as CK5 and CK17, vimentin, muscle-specific actin, myosin, P63, smooth muscle actin, and calponin. Although glial fibrillary acidic protein is positive in myoepithelial cells of PA, it is only focally positive in ACC. S100 protein has been reported positive in most ACC cases. Also, cKit (CD117) has been positive in most ACC cases, especially the solid variant, whereas P53 is expressed in low levels, except in the solid variant. Finally, like other salivary gland tumors, ACC usually expresses mucin 1.

Few studies have revealed cytogenetic aberrations, including translocation in chromosome 9p13-23 and deletion in 9p21. Also, few molecular studies revealed genetic abnormalities such as overexpression of gene sox-4 and AP-2α.

11.4 CYTOLOGIC DIFFERENTIAL DIAGNOSIS

Table 11.2 lists some common differences for major differential cytologic diagnoses.

11.4.1 Pleomorphic Adenoma

The aspirate of pleomorphic adenoma shows small fragments of chondro myxoid stroma and cell clusters with peripheral spindle cells streaming into myxofibrillary stroma. This is the most difficult differential because both tumors display a cellular aspirate of bland small uniform cells with cylinders or gland-cribriform structures and hyaline globules. However, hyaline globules are variably staining, feathery, irregular, and myxofibrillary in PA, whereas they are homogenous dense, rounded, nonfibrillary, and intensely metachromatic on Diff-Quik stain in ACC. They are also few and small in PA, whereas they are diffuse and many in ACC. Also, small fragments of connective tissue may be embedded in the hyaline material in ACC, whereas the presence of single spindle cells in the hyaline material is more suggestive of PA. The characteristic fibrillary chondromyxoid stroma and the plasmacytoid and spindled myoepithelial cells in PA are absent in ACC. Furthermore, squamous cell differentiation can be observed in PA but not in ACC. Also, clinical evidence of nerve invasion, such as pain (sharp pain during the FNAB procedure is characteristic) or paralysis, or the presence of diffuse cytologic atypia (including hyperchromasia, coarse chromatin, and prominent nucleoli) usually indicates malignancy (Table 11.3).

TABLE 11.2. Major Cytologic differential diagnoses	
	Clues to make the distinction
Pleomorphic adenoma	Hyaline stroma is irregular, feathery, variably staining, and myxofibrillary Single spindle cells blends at the periphery of hyaline material Squamous metaplasia Chondromyxoid stroma, plasmacytoid, and spindle myoepithelial cells Uncommon cellular atypia, nucleoli, or hyperchromasia
Basal cell adenoma	Cells are more uniform, smaller, and cohesive No cell overlapping No atypia or mitoses, or nucleoli No clinical signs of nerve damage No squamous or basosquamous differentiation or tumor necrosis
Trabecular adenoma	Smaller hyaline material Cells are small, uniform, and more bland
Epithelial-myoepithelial carcinoma	Also has dual cell population Myoepithelial cells are conspicuous, larger, and polygonal with clear cytoplasm and round nuclei Usually, IHC is not helpful
Acinic cell carcinoma	Predominance of cells with abundant granular cytoplasm and absence of thick hyalinized material
Polymorphous low-grade adenocarcinoma (PLGA)	Cells are uniform epithelial with round vesicular-achromatic nuclei and eosinophilic cytoplasm No reactivity of smooth muscle actin, myosin, and calponin CEA, EMA, and S100 protein are more intensely and diffusely positive in PLGA

11.4.2   Monomorphic Adenoma (Basal Cell Adenoma)

Aspirates of the solid variant of ACC can look similar to those of monomorphic adenoma. In contrast to basal cell adenoma, the solid variant of ACC often shows a cellular specimen with overlapping, larger, and more variable nuclei, mitoses, and small nucleoli. The differential here is critical and can be difficult to identify, especially when hyaline cores or globules are absent. As a general rule, the presence of necrosis, clearly visible nucleoli, irregular nuclei, and abnormal coarse chromatin favors ACC (solid variant). Clinical nerve damage (pain or paralysis), absence of squamous or

TABLE 11.3. Aspiration cytology of adenoid cystic carcinoma versus pleomorphic adenoma		
	Adenoid cystic carcinoma	Pleomorphic adenoma
Architecture	Cohesive clusters, cords, glands, or cribriform structures	Trabeculae, glands, ducts, or cohesive clusters. Single plasmacytoid (hyaline cells); spindle or stellate cells embedded in stroma
Epithelial cells	Small uniform basoloid with round–oval nuclei	Small round–oval with round bland nuclei
Myoepithelial cells	Mostly single	Single, plasmacytoid (hyaline cells)
Nucleoli	Maybe prominent	No
Mucoid stromal substance	Hyaline globules: dense homogenous rounded spherical	Myxofibrillary, feathery, and irregular
Squamous metaplasia	Sometimes	No
Clinical nerve damage	Maybe	No

basosquamous differentiation, anaplastic or significant cellular atypia, and minimal vascularity in the stroma all favor ACC. The cells are also more cohesive in monomorphic adenoma than in ACC.

11.4.3   Trabecular Adenoma (Membranous Variant of Basal Cell Adenoma)

Trabecular adenoma is a controversial tumor believed to be a subvariant of monomorphic adenoma that closely resembles ACC with the presence of small, uniform basaloid cells and hyaline globules. However, the hyaline material is usually small in trabecular adenoma, whereas it is more variable in size and outline, including large branching forms, in ACC. In practice, the distinction between the two entities can be very difficult to assess.

11.4.4   Small Cell Carcinoma

Small cell carcinoma also may be considered in this situation, but the cells of ACC are uniform, small, and bland compared with those of small cell carcinoma

11.4.5 Acinic Cell Carcinoma

The main indicator of acinic cell carcinoma is the distinctive predominance of tumor cells with an abundant granular cytoplasm.

11.4.6 Polymorphous Low-Grade Adenocarcinoma (PLGA)

Polymorphous low-grade adenocarcinoma (PLGA) may be confused most often with the cribriform or tubular variants of ACC. The differential, however, is important because of different biologic behavior. PLGA is extremely rare in major salivary glands and most often involves the oral minor salivary glands. Although the cells of ACC tend to be uniform with pale–clear cytoplasm and hyperchromatic angular nuclei, the cells of PLGA are uniform epithelial with round vesicular–achromatic nuclei and eosinophilic cytoplasm. Immunohistochemistry is useful with the reactivity of smooth muscle actin, myosin, and calponin in ACC (myoepithelial cells) but not in PLGA. Also, CEA, EMA, and S100 protein have been reported more intensely and diffusely positive in PLGA.

11.4.7 Epithelial-Myoepithelial Carcinoma (EMC)

Epithelial-myoepithelial carcinoma, as the name indicates, also has a dual cell population. In the aspirate slides of this tumor, the myoepithelial cells are conspicuously larger and polygonal with clear cytoplasm and round nuclei. The cells of ACC are small, basaloid, and bland. IHC generally is not helpful in the differential diagnosis.

11.4.8 Adenocarcinoma

In adenocarcinoma, the hyaline globules are small droplets, whereas those of ACC are large cylindrical or branching thick structures. Mucous-producing adenocarcinoma also can resemble ACC.

11.5 PROGNOSIS AND TREATMENT

The prognosis is generally poor because of incomplete or difficult surgical resection and frequency of metastases, which is dependent on the site of involvement and is most common in the palate.

Although it has an indolent growth, it is well known for its persistence, frequent recurrences, and late metastasis. Overall, patients have a good 5-year survival rate and a poor 10–20-year survival rate. Different biologic behaviors and clinical courses are related to growth patterns, with the solid pattern having the worst prognosis. However, because of the common mixture of growth patterns, grading of tumors is sometimes difficult or inaccurate. The clinical stage seems to be a better predictor of clinical outcome than histologic grading. Tumor size and regional lymph node metastasis are associated with a poor prognosis. Some studies showed that the presence and extent of perineural invasion probably is associated with treatment failures. Distant metastasis to the lungs and bones, which often develop in the absence of regional lymph node metastasis, has a poor prognosis.

The treatment of choice is wide or radical excision followed by post-operative radiation. Chemotherapy has a limited role and has been reserved only for advanced tumors or as a palliative option. The recent reports of c-kitt (CD 117) positivity in ACC indicate possible benefits from targeted gene therapy by the tyrosine kinase inhibitors such as imitinib or sunatinib.

RECOMMENDED READINGS

Al-Khafaji BM, Afify AM. Salivary gland fine needle aspiration using the ThinPrep technique: diagnostic accuracy, cytologic artifacts and pitfalls. Acta Cytol 2001;45:567–574.

Al-Khafaji BM, Nestok BR, Katz RL. Fine-needle aspiration of 154 parotid masses with histologic correlation: ten-year experience at the University of Texas M. D. Anderson Cancer Center. Cancer 1998;84:153–159.

Bianchi B, Copelli C, Cocchi R, Ferrari S, Pederneschi N, Sesenna E. Adenoid cystic carcinoma of intraoral minor salivary glands. Oral Oncol 2008;44:1026–1031.

Bibbo M. Fine needle aspiration of salivary glands. Acta Cytol 2009;53:367–368.

Cajulis RS, Gokaslan ST, Yu GH, Frias-Hidvegi D. Fine needle aspiration biopsy of the salivary glands. A five-year experience with emphasis on diagnostic pitfalls. Acta Cytol 1997;41:1412–1420.

Daneshbod Y, Daneshbod K, Khademi B. Diagnostic difficulties in the interpretation of fine needle aspirate samples in salivary lesions: diagnostic pitfalls revisited. Acta Cytol 2009;53:53–70.

DeMay R. The Art and Science of Cytopathology. Volume II, Aspiration Cytology. Chicago (IL): ASCP Press; 1996. p 676–679.

Ellis GL, Auclair PL. Tumors of the Salivary Glands. AFIP Atlas of Tumor Pathology, 4th Series, Fascicle 9. Silver Spring (MD): ARP Press; 2008: p 225–246.

Eveson J. Malignant neoplasms of the salivary glands. In: Thompson LD, Goldblum JR, editors. Head and Neck Pathology, Foundation in Diagnostic Pathology. Amsterdam (The Netherlands): Churchill Livingston-Elsevier; 2006. p 339–345.

Hughes JH, Volk EE, Wilbur DC, Cytopathology Resource Committee, College of American Pathologists. Pitfalls in salivary gland fine-needle aspiration cytology: lessons from the College of American Pathologists Interlaboratory Comparison Program in nongynecologic cytology. Arch Pathol Lab Med 2005;129:26–31.

Khafif A, Anavi Y, Haviv J, Fienmesser R, Calderon S, Marshak G. Adenoid cystic carcinoma of the salivary glands: a 20-year review with long-term follow-up. Ear Nose Throat J 2005;84:662, 664–667.

Klijanienko J, Vielh P. Fine-needle sampling of salivary gland lesions. III. Cytologic and histologic correlation of 75 cases of adenoid cystic carcinoma: review and experience at the Institute Curie with emphasis on cytologic pitfalls. Diagn Cytopathol 1997;17:36–41.

Nagel H, Hotze HJ, Laskawi R, Chilla R, Droese M. Cytologic diagnosis of adenoid cystic carcinoma of salivary glands. Diagn Cytopathol 1999;20:358–366.

Rajwanshi A, Gupta K, Gupta N, Shukla R, Srinivasan R, Nijhawan R, Vasishta R. Fine-needle aspiration cytology of salivary glands: diagnostic pitfalls—revisited. Diagn Cytopathol 2006;34:580–584.

Schindler S, Nayar R, Dutra J, Bedrossian CW. Diagnostic challenges in aspiration cytology of the salivary glands. Semin Diagn Pathol 2001;18:124–146.

Stanley MW, Horwitz CA, Rollins SD, Powers CN, Bardales RH, Korourain S, Stern SJ. Basal cell (monomorphic) and minimally pleomorphic adenomas of the salivary·glands. Distinction from the solid (anaplastic) type of adenoid cystic carcinoma in fine-needle aspiration. Am J Clin Pathol 1996;106: 35–41.

Stewart CJ, MacKenzie K, McGarry GW, Mowat A. Fine-needle aspiration cytology of salivary gland: a review of 341 cases. Diagn Cytopathol 2000;22:139–146.

Zhang S, Bao R, Bagby J, Abreo F. Fine needle aspiration of salivary glands: 5-year experience from a single academic center. Acta Cytol 2009;53:375–382.

CHAPTER 12

ONCOCYTOMA

JAY K. WASMAN, MD and FADI W. ABDUL-KARIM, MD

12.1 INTRODUCTION

Oncocytes develop from the accumulation of large numbers of abnormal mitochondria within epithelial cells resulting in cytoplasmic enlargement with granularity and a low nuclear cytoplasmic ratio. Although this process can occur in many types of epithelial cells, oncocytic change within salivary glands is extremely common and seems to be an age-related phenomenon. Whether this change occurs because of an intracellular abnormality or in response to external stimuli has not been defined clearly. The term "oncocytosis" is used when oncocytic change is prominent. Oncocytosis can occur in either diffuse or nodular forms.

The 2005 World Health Organization Classification of Tumours: Pathology and Genetics of Head and Neck Tumours defines oncocytoma as a "benign tumour of salivary gland origin composed exclusively of large epithelial cells with characteristic bright eosinophilic granular cytoplasm (oncocytic cells)." Separation of nodular oncocytosis (nodular oncocytic metaplasia) from oncocytoma may be difficult; however, when an oncocytic proliferation is circumscribed, at least partially encapsulated, and large enough to be clinically detectable, it is classified best as an oncocytoma.

12.2 CLINICAL FEATURES

Oncocytomas comprise approximately 1% of all salivary gland neoplasms. They occur most commonly in the sixth through eighth decades with a mean age of 58 years. There is no sex predilection. Approximately 84% of major

Salivary Gland Cytology: A Color Atlas, Edited by Mousa A. Al-Abbadi
Copyright © 2011 Wiley-Blackwell

salivary gland oncocytomas occur in the parotid, with the remainder in the submandibular gland. Lesions developing in the minor salivary glands are uncommon, but they do occur. Parotid gland oncocytoma most often presents as a painless mass.

There are no clear etiologies for most oncocytomas. Occasional oncocytoma patients, however, have a history of prior radiation therapy or prolonged radiation exposure to the head and neck. These patients present at a younger age as compared with the nonradiation-exposed individuals.

12.3 CYTOLOGIC FEATURES WITH HISTOLOGIC CORRELATES

12.3.1 Gross Features

Oncocytomas are well circumscribed, solid, tan-brown nodules without evidence of hemorrhage or necrosis. They are encapsulated at least partially and typically measure 3–4 cm, although lesions can range up to 7 cm.

12.3.2 Cytologic Features

Fine needle aspiration biopsies of oncocytomas yield cellular specimens. The smears contain abundant large cells present as individual cells, clusters, papillary fragments, and sheets (Figure 12.1). The oncocytic cells have abundant granular cytoplasm with a low nuclear cytoplasmic ratio and distinct cytoplasmic borders (Figures 12.2–12.5). On alcohol-fixed, Papinicolaou-stained slides, the cytoplasm is blue-gray to orange-pink and granular (Figures 12.2, 12.3, and 12.5). On air-dried, Romanowsky-stained slides, the cytoplasm appears blue and without observable granules (Figure 12.4). The nuclei of oncocytic cells are round to oval, centrally placed, and may contain variably sized nucleoli (Figures 12.2–12.5). Some oncocytomas may show nuclear enlargement with vesicular chromatin. Naked nuclei representing isolated oncocytes usually are observed in the background (Figure 12.1). In tumors with a clear cell component, the tumor cells contain abundant optically clear (Papinicolaou stain) or microvacuolated (Romanowsky stain) cytoplasm. Smears from oncocytomas typically are devoid of inflammatory cells.

12.3.3 Histopathologic Features

Oncocytomas are well-circumscribed/encapsulated lesions that can have solid, trabecular, and/or acinar architectural patterns (Figure 12.6). Occasional tumors are partially or predominantly cystic. Oncocytes have abundant eosinophilic granular cytoplasm with centrally placed, oval, and vesicular nuclei that may contain single or multiple prominent nucleoli (Figure 12.7). Cells containing eosinophilic cytoplasm with pyknotic nuclei

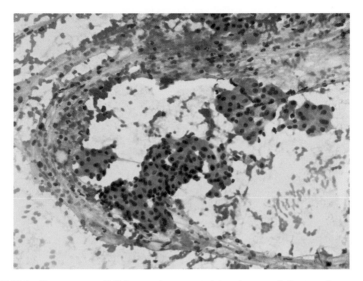

FIGURE 12.1. Oncocytoma. Cellular specimen containing sheets and clusters of oncocytes and scattered naked nuclei (Papanicolaou ×200).

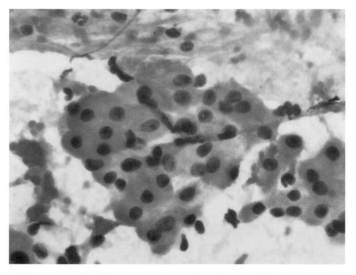

FIGURE 12.2. Oncocytoma. Oncocytes contain abundant, granular pink-red cytoplasm with uniform, round-to-oval nuclei and occasional variably prominent nucleoli (Papanicolaou ×600).

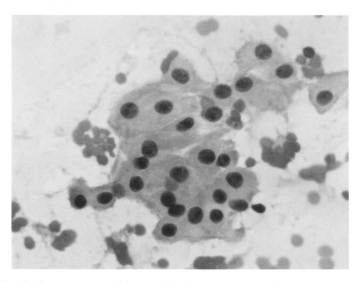

FIGURE 12.3. Oncocytoma. In this example, the oncocytes' abundant granular cytoplasm is gray-blue, rather than pink-red, as shown in Figures 12.1 and 12.2 (Papanicolaou ×600).

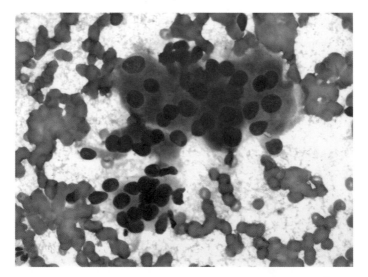

FIGURE 12.4. Oncocytoma. Oncocytes contain abundant, waxy blue cytoplasm without observable granules and uniform round-to-oval nuclei (Romanowsky ×600). Courtesy of C. Michael, University of Michigan Health System, Ann Arbor, MI.

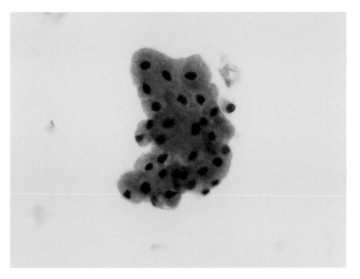

FIGURE 12.5. Oncocytoma. In this liquid-based preparation, the oncocytes contain abundant, granular gray–blue-to-orange cytoplasm with small, uniform round-to-oval nuclei (Papanicolaou ×600).

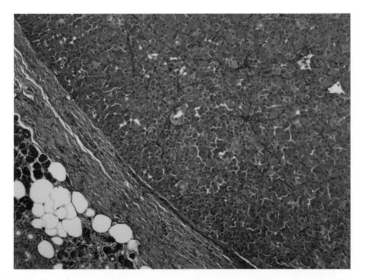

FIGURE 12.6. Oncocytoma. Sheets and nests of oncocytic cells are separated from normal parotid gland parenchyma (lower left) by a well-defined fibrous capsule (hematoxylin and eosin ×100).

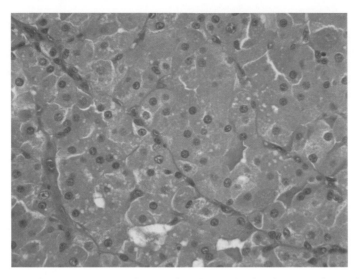

FIGURE 12.7. Oncocytoma. Nests of oncocytic cells contain abundant, granular, eosinophilic cytoplasm. Uniform round-to-oval nuclei are placed centrally and contain occasional variably prominent nucleoli (hematoxylin and eosin ×400).

also are observed. In addition, some oncocytomas contain clear cells, either intermixed with the typical oncocytes or as the predominant cell type. Mitotic figures only are observed rarely. The tumor cell mitochondria stain with phosphotungstic acid hematoxylin (PTAH). By immunohisto-chemistry, oncocytoma cells stain with cytokeratins and antimitochondrial antibody.

12.4 CYTOLOGIC DIFFERENTIAL DIAGNOSIS

The main cytologic differential diagnosis for oncocytoma is oncocytosis, Warthin's tumor, and oncocytic carcinoma. Oncocytosis is distinguished from oncocytoma based on the architectural features and distribution of the oncocytic cells within the parotid gland rather than by cytologic features. Oncocytoma is separated from a Warthin's tumor by the absence of a lymphoid component and of a cystic change in oncocytoma. The oncocytic cellular component is indistinguishable in the two lesions.

Oncocytic carcinoma typically shows atypia, pleomorphism, and mitotic activity to a much greater extent than oncocytomas (Figures 12.8–12.11). Some cases of oncocytic carcinoma, however, can show features identical to those of oncocytoma. These cases require the demonstration of invasive growth (angioinvasion or capsular invasion) on histopathologic sections to establish a diagnosis of oncocytic carcinoma.

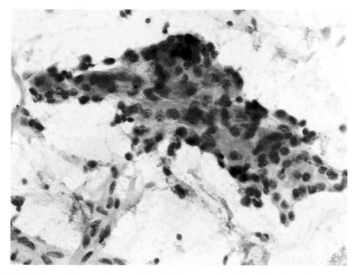

FIGURE 12.8. Oncocytic carcinoma. Sheet of oncocytic cells with abundant, granular gray-blue cytoplasm. Nuclei are crowded, with some enlargement, vesicular chromatin, and scattered small nucleoli (Papanicolaou ×400). Courtesy of T. Elsheikh, Ball Memorial Hospital, Muncie, IN.

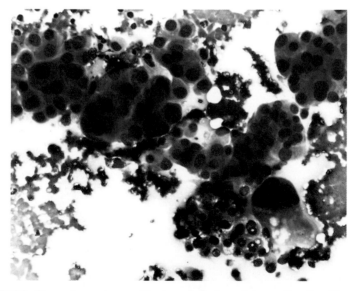

FIGURE 12.9. Oncocytic carcinoma. Sheets and clusters of oncocytic cells with gray-blue, waxy cytoplasm. Nuclei are crowded, and the nuclear cytoplasmic ratio is higher than that observed in oncocytoma specimens. Occasional scattered markedly enlarged pleomorphic nuclei are identified (MCG ×200). Courtesy of J.Klijanienko, Institut Curie, Paris, France.

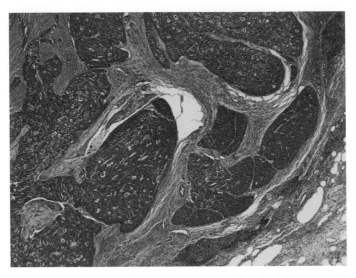

FIGURE 12.10. Oncocytic carcinoma. In contrast to the well-defined fibrous capsule observed in oncocytomas, oncocytic carcinoma demonstrates an invasive growth pattern with desmoplastic stroma (hematoxylin and eosin ×40).

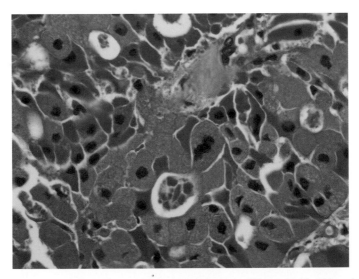

FIGURE 12.11. Oncocytic carcinoma, higher magnification of Figure 12.10. Although the cells retain the characteristic abundant, eosinophilic, and granular cytoplasm, significant nuclear pleomorphism is present in scattered cells (hematoxylin and eosin ×600).

TABLE 12.1. Key diagnostic features of oncocytoma
• Cellular specimen
• Large epithelial cells with a low N/C ratio present individually and in cohesive clusters and sheets
• Cells contain abundant PTAH positive granular cytoplasm
• Nuclei are round to oval and may contain variably sized nucleoli
• Lymphoid and/or cystic components are absent

Oncocytic changes may be observed in some cases of pleomorphic adenoma, acinic cell carcinoma, and mucoepidermoid carcinoma. Occasional pleomorphic adenomas show extensive oncocytic metaplasia; in these instances, separation from oncocytoma depends on identifying the typical chondromyxoid stroma observed in pleomorphic adenomas. Acinic cell carcinomas may show considerable cytologic overlap with oncocytoma, making the distinction difficult. Like oncocytoma, the neoplastic cells in acinic cell carcinoma contain abundant cytoplasm that can be vacuolated or coarsely granular. Acinic cell carcinoma tumor cells, however, often are present in acinar structures, though solid sheets and papillary formations also can be present. Although the nuclei are typically bland with features similar to normal acinar cells, varying degrees of atypia can be observed. Cell-block material, if available, may be helpful, as the cytoplasmic granules in oncocytes stain with PTAH and are negative for periodic acid-Schif (PAS) with diastase, whereas the cytoplasmic granules in acinic cell carcinoma show the opposite staining pattern. The oncocytic variant of mucoepidermoid carcinoma may be difficult to separate from an oncocytoma; however, mucus cells are present in mucoepidermoid carcinoma and only are observed rarely in oncocytoma.

The cytologic differential diagnosis of the clear cell variant of oncocytoma is broad, as several salivary gland neoplasms can consist, in part or entirely, of clear cells. These neoplasms include clear cell adenocarcinoma, acinic cell carcinoma, myoepithelioma, myoepithelial carcinoma, epithelial-myoepithelial carcinoma, mucoepidermoid carcinoma, and metastatic clear cell carcinoma. In general, the presence of oncocytic cells admixed with clear cells favors oncocytoma. A PTAH stain performed on cell block material may be extremely useful in separating clear cell oncocytoma from other entities containing clear cells. Table 12.2 summarizes the differential diagnosis and gives clues to make the distinctions.

12.5 TREATMENT OF CHOICE AND PROGNOSIS

The treatment of choice for an oncocytoma is complete surgical resection. The prognosis is very good with local recurrence occurring in up to 10%

TABLE 12.2. Differential diagnosis of oncocytoma

	Clues to Make the Distinction
Warthin's tumor	Warthin's tumor has a lymphoid component and often a cystic background; oncocytic component is indistinguishable
Oncocytic carcinoma	Oncocytic carcinoma usually exhibits significant atypia, pleomorphism, and mitotic activity; rare examples may show a lack of these features and are not separable from oncocytoma by cytology
Pleomorphic adenoma with oncocytic metaplasia	Chondro-myxoid stroma should be found in pleomorphic adenoma and should be absent in oncocytoma
Mucoepidermoid carcinoma, oncocytic variant	Oncocytic variant of mucoepidermoid carcinoma contains scattered mucus cells; mucus cells only are observed rarely in oncytoma
Acinic cell carcinoma	PTAH positive cytoplasmic granules are present in oncocytoma, whereas PAS positive, diastase resistant granules are present in acinic cell carcinoma. Acinic cell carcinoma often retains acinar architecture
Clear cell neoplasms	Unlike other clear cell neoplasms, clear cell oncocytomas usually contain a component of typical oncocytes; PTAH stain of cytoplasmic granules also may aid in the distinction

of cases. The presence of oncocytic changes in other entities do not affect their prognosis.

RECOMMENDED READINGS

Abdul-Karim FW, Weaver MG. Needle aspiration cytology of an oncocytic carcinoma of the parotid gland. Diagn Cytopathol 1991;7:420–422.

Brandwein MS, Huvos AG. Oncocytic tumors of the major salivary glands: a study of 68 cases with follow-up of 44 patients. Am J Surg Pathol 1991;15:514–528.

Ellis GL, Auclair PL. Tumors of the Salivary Glands. AFIP Atlas of Tumor Pathology, 4th Series, Fascicle 9. Silver Spring (MD): ARP Press; 2008. p 100–109.

Huvos AG. Oncocytoma. In: Barnes L, Eveson JW, Reichart P, Sidransky D, editors. Pathology and Genetics of Head and Neck Tumours. World Health Organization Classification of Tumours. Lyon (France): IARC Press; 2005. p 266.

Krane JF, Faquin WC. Salivary gland. In: Cibas ES, Ducatman BS, editors. Cytology: Diagnostic Principles and Clinical correlates. 3rd ed. Philadelphia (PA): Saunders Elsevier; 2009. p 301–303.

Odile D, Blaney S, Hearp M. Parotid gland fine-needle aspiration cytology: an approach to differential diagnosis. Diagn Cytopathol 2007;35:47–56.

Verma K, Kapila K. Salivary gland tumors with a prominent oncocytic component: cytologic findings and differential diagnosis of oncocytomas and Warthin's tumor on fine needle aspirates. Acta Cytol 2003;47:221–226.

Wakely PE. Oncocytic and oncocyte-like lesions of the head and neck. Ann Diagn Pathol 2008;12:222–230.

CHAPTER 13

MYOEPITHELIOMA AND RELATED LESIONS

PAMELA PAPAS, MD and MOMIN T. SIDDIQUI, MD

13.1 INTRODUCTION

Myoepithelial cells (of ectodermal origin and mesodermal functionality), normal constituent cells of ductal structures in major and minor salivary glands and other organs, are modified cellular elements with both epithelial and myocontractile properties. They are component cells in a variety of salivary gland neoplasms both benign and malignant; they are present, for example, in pleomorphic adenoma, adenoid cystic carcinoma, and terminal duct carcinoma, which are entities previously reviewed. Uncommonly, in a few neoplasms, myoepithelial cells are the exclusive or predominant ($\geq 95\%$) cellular population, and tumors of this type comprise $< 5\%$ of salivary gland tumors, thereby defining myoepithelioma and its malignant counterpart, malignant myoepithelioma (myoepithelial carcinoma); this chapter also will include the closely related epithelial-myoepithelial carcinoma. Most reviewers agree that myoepithelioma is more than likely a monomorphic variant (exclusively/predominantly comprising myoepithelial cells) of pleomorphic adenoma lacking ductal differentiation. It is noteworthy that many typical salivary gland neoplasms, including those under current discussion, may occur in nonsalivary gland locations and may be, for example, of breast, bronchial gland, skin, prostate (benign myoepithelioma), and rarely, even maxillary sinus (malignant myoepithelial counterpart) origin.

Salivary Gland Cytology: A Color Atlas, Edited by Mousa A. Al-Abbadi
Copyright © 2011 Wiley-Blackwell

13.2 MYOEPITHELIOMA

13.2.1 Clinical Features

Clinical features encompassing age and gender distribution are not surprisingly similar to those of pleomorphic adenoma, considering that most agree these tumors represent monomorphic variants of mixed tumors. They occur typically in the major and minor salivary glands with roughly equal gender predilection, a broad age range of 9–85 years of age, and an average age of 44 years. These tumors tend to be slow growing and are usually asymptomatic.

Myoepitheliomas may comprise one or more than one morphologic cell type. Most spindle and clear cell subtypes occur in the parotid gland, whereas the plasmacytoid/hyaline variant is encountered more commonly in minor salivary glands, particularly in the palate.

Though most myoepitheliomas are benign, the spindle cell and particularly the clear cell subtypes have demonstrated malignant variants, demonstrating invasive characteristics and significant cytological atypia. Spindle cell differentiation correlates with aggressive behavior. It has been suggested that the clear cell variant be regarded as potentially malignant as local recurrences, lymph node metastases, and tumor-related deaths have been described. Hyaline/plasmacytoid varieties tend to behave in a benign fashion. Malignant myoepitheliomas may develop de novo or via malignant transformation of pleomorphic adenoma/basal cell adenoma and occasionally in a benign myoepithelioma.

13.2.2 Cytological Features and Histological Correlate

Benign myoepithelial neoplasms may be divided into the following morphologic cellular subtypes: spindle cell, plasmacytoid/hyaline, epithelioid, and clear cell types, which may occur in pure form or in various proportions in a single neoplasm. The fine needle aspirates of these neoplasms may be cellular.

Single cells or loosely cohesive groups of cells are present with variable features depending on the predominating cell type. Typically, there are loosely cohesive fusiform/spindle cells, often stellate, which possess delicate, ill-defined cytoplasm and elongate nuclei with fine chromatin and inconspicuous/small nucleoli (Figure 13.1). Epithelioid cells possess better-defined cytoplasmic borders with round to ovoid nuclei and evenly distributed fine chromatin. There is a lack of honeycombed sheets of epithelial cells and a lack of chondromyxoid matrix in contrast to pleomorphic adenoma (Figure 13.2).

Plasmacytoid/hyaline cells are endowed with eosinophilic, dense, and nongranular cytoplasm as a result of prekeratin intermediate filaments imparting a hyaline quality to the fibrillar or glassy cytoplasm, and these cells possess eccentric, sometimes pleomorphic nuclei occasionally accompanied by rare mitoses. Stromal elements are characteristically lacking. Clear cells of the clear

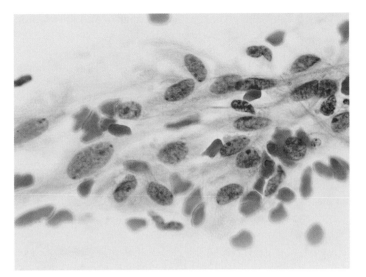

FIGURE 13.1. Myoepithelial cells are wispy aggregates of fusiform cells with frayed cytoplasmic borders, spindly nuclei, fine chromatin, occasional nucleoli, and minimal cytological atypia (Papanicolaou stain 400×). Courtesy of R.M. DeMay, M.D., University of Chicago Medical Center, Chicago, Illinois.

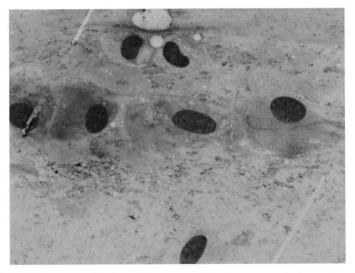

FIGURE 13.2. Plasmacytoid/hyaline cells possess moderate amounts of nongranular cytoplasm with eccentric (sometimes pleomorphic) nuclei. Stromal elements are not present. (Diff-Quik stain 400×). Courtesy of R.M. DeMay, M.D., University of Chicago Medical Center, Chicago, Illinois.

cell variant possess cells with glycogen-rich cytoplasm and are accompanied by nuclei with evenly distributed fine chromatin. The key diagnostic features are summarized in Table 13.1.

Histologically, most examples in the parotid gland are encapsulated, whereas those in minor salivary glands are unencapsulated. As previously mentioned, similarities to pleomorphic adenoma are described; however, there is predominance or a nearly exclusive population of myoepithelial cells comprising myoepitheliomas (Figure 13.3).

TABLE 13.1. Key diagnostic features of myoepithelioma

- Cellular aspirates
- Exclusive, predominant, or variable mix of spindle, epithelioid, plasmacytoid (hyaline), and/or clear cells
- Typically consist of single cells and loosely cohesive sheets of spindle cells with minimal cytological atypia and frayed cytoplasmic borders
- Bipolar bare myoepithelial nuclei may be present in background
- Nuclei possess fine chromatin with small/indistinct nucleoli
- Lack of stromal elements
- Monomorphic population of cells
- Few to rare mitotic figures

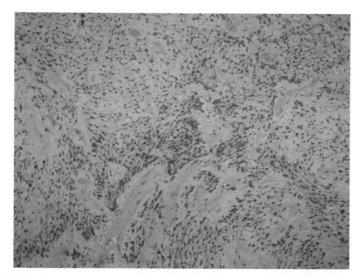

FIGURE 13.3. Histologic section of an exclusive population of myoepithelial cells with bland morphologic features. (hematoxylin and eosin stain 100×). Courtesy of R.M. DeMay, M.D., University of Chicago Medical Center, Chicago, Illinois.

13.2.3 Differential Diagnoses

Spindle cell myoepitheliomas overlap morphologically with other spindle cells tumors, including those of smooth muscle, Schwann cell (either of which may show Verocay bodies), or fibroblast origin. Immunohistochemical staining usually aids in this distinction.

Plasmacytoid myoepitheliomas superficially may resemble plasmacytomas though electrophoresis, kappa and lambda immunostaining, a lack of distinctive nuclear cytomorphologic features (clockface chromatin), and a lack of perinuclear hof aid in the exclusion of plasmacytomas.

Epithelioid myoepitheliomas may resemble other salivary gland neoplasms including mucoepidermoid carcinoma, acinic cell carcinoma, basal cell adenoma, polymorphous low-grade adenocarcinoma, as well as tumors metastatic to the involved site. Clinical, morphologic, and immunohistochemical correlation is essential.

Clear cell myoepithelioma, which demonstrates glycogen on periodic acid-Schiff (PAS) stain, requires distinction from other tumors with clear cell features, including sebaceous neoplasms (which demonstrate fat), mucoepidermoid carcinoma (which demonstrates mucin), acinic cell carcinoma (which is typically negative for special histochemical staining properties), and clear cell change in oncocytic tumors. Other differential diagnostic possibilities in appropriate clinical settings may include metastatic renal cell carcinoma (which demonstrates glycogen and immunohistochemically is positive for vimentin and CD10, and is negative for HMW-CK and carcinoembryonic antigen [CEA]), and clear cell carcinoma and not otherwise specified (NOS)/hyalanizing clear cell carcinoma usually present in the oral cavity (a diagnosis of exclusion of other neoplasms), which notably include conspicuous fibrohyaline stroma. Epithelial-myoepithelial carcinoma may enter the differential diagnosis; however, typically, the characteristic dual cell population is evident. Malignant myoepithelioma may bear cytomorphologic resemblance, though increased nuclear atypia and the clinical presentation may raise suspicion for this entity. Histologic follow-up of epithelial-myoepithelial carcinoma or malignant myoepithelioma will present infiltrative foci supportive of their malignant nature. The differential diagnosis and clues to make the distinctions are summarized in Table 13.2.

The immunoprofile of myoepithelial cells often is employed to distinguish the aforementioned differential diagnostic possibilities; myoepithelial cells are typically positive for cytokeratin, S-100, calponin, glial fibrillary acidic protein (GFAP), vimentin, smooth muscle actin (SMA), and smooth muscle myosin-heavy chain (SMM-HC) and can help distinguish myoepithelial cells from other cell types. The lack of both chondromyxoid matrix and sheets of epithelial cells is helpful in favoring a myoepithelial-rich neoplasm (vs. a pleomorphic adenoma, for example). Nonetheless, sampling discrepancies must be considered. The lack of clinical consequence in this distinction

TABLE 13.2. Differential diagnosis of myoepithelioma	
	Clues to make the distinction
Pleomorphic adenoma	Varying proportions of epithelial (honeycomb sheets) and loose aggregates of myoepithelial cells present Chondromyxoid matrix present Epithelial and myoepithelial cell immunoprofiles
Spindle cell tumors	Spindle cell population present Spindle cell immunoprofile
Epithelial/epithelioid tumors	Epithelial/epithelioid cell population present Epithelial cell immunoprofile
Clear cell tumors	Clear cell population present; depending on origin, may demonstrate fat, mucin, or glycogen May present site-specific immunoprofile (i.e., renal cell carcinoma [RCC] positive by immunohistochemistry in clear cell renal cell carcinoma)
Plasmacytoma	Plasma cell population present Nuclear clock face chromatin Granular eosinophilic cytoplasm κ/λ monoclonality demonstrated; appropriate protein electrophoresis pattern in clinical setting

supports value in offering a descriptive diagnosis for fine needle aspirates of myoepithelial-predominant neoplasms, offering an appropriate differential diagnosis of myoepithelioma, myoepithelial-rich pleomorphic adenoma, and pleomorphic adenoma sampling myoepithelial cells.

A suggested practical bottom line diagnosis, "myoepithelial cell-rich neoplasm," accompanied by a brief discussion of differential diagnoses and results of immunohistochemical studies if available (although cell blocks may be variably cellular) may serve the clinician adequately, prompting appropriate surgical intervention.

13.2.4 Treatment and Prognosis

Surgical excision with clear margins is the standard of care for benign myoepitheliomas, though they may recur nonetheless. Spindle cell variants may behave more aggressively and warrant meticulous surgically free margins.

13.3 MALIGNANT MYOEPITHELIOMA (MYOEPITHELIAL CARCINOMA)

13.3.1 Clinical Features

Malignant myoepithelioma, the malignant counterpart of benign myoepithelioma—a tumor of older adults (mean age of 55 years)—occurs most commonly in the parotid gland, less frequently in the submandibular gland and minor salivary glands, and with equal incidence in males and females. These tumors comprise <2% of salivary gland carcinomas and usually present as a painless mass. Recurrences are not unusual, though metastases are uncommon. Locally destructive behavior is typical. Approximately 60–70% develop in benign mixed tumors (carcinoma ex pleomorphic adenoma) or benign myoepitheliomas, and the remainder develop de novo.

13.3.2 Cytological Features and Histological Correlate

Cytological aspirates are typically cellular to hypercellular and comprise single cells and large tissue fragments. These fragments appear three-dimensional with considerable nuclear overlapping and crowding. Metachromatic stromal fragments occasionally are observed to be intermixed with the neoplastic cells (Figure 13.4). Usually, the neoplastic cells are spindly with variable amounts of wispy pale cytoplasm and frayed cytoplasmic borders. Scattered epithelioid, plasmacytoid, and clear cells may be present. The nuclei range from oval to elongate to spindle-shaped and vary

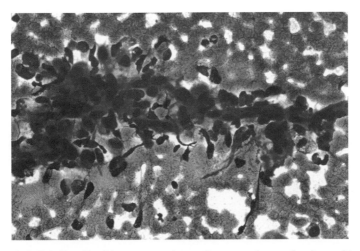

FIGURE 13.4. Spindle cells with scant metachromatic stroma also can be observed in aspirate samples. (Diff-Quik stain 400×). Courtesy of R.M. DeMay, M.D., University of Chicago Medical Center, Chicago, Illinois.

considerably in size. Nuclear chromatin is coarsely granular and nucleoli are evident (Figure 13.5). Binucleate and multinucleate tumor cells as well as rare mitotic figures may accompany the aforementioned uninucleate tumor cells. Cytological atypia, pleomorphism, necrosis, and mitotic activity, present in some though not all cases, raise suspicion for malignancy, a concern that requires histological confirmation. Proliferative activity, assessed immunohistochemically by Ki-67, has been suggested to predict malignancy in cases with greater than 10% labeling. Significant proliferative activity, marked pleomorphism, and p53 immunoreactivity by immunohistochemistry on cellblock material portend aggressive clinical behavior. The key diagnostic features are summarized in Table 13.3.

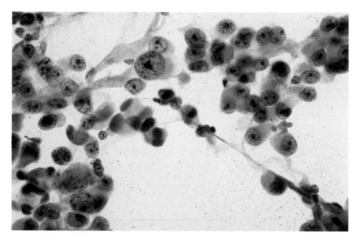

FIGURE 13.5. Aggregates of cells show a relatively haphazard arrangement of cells with worrisome nuclear features; coarse chromatin and nucleoli are noted. (Papanicolaou stain 640×). Courtesy of S. Kini, M.D., Henry Ford Hospital, Detroit, Michigan.

TABLE 13.3. Key diagnostic features of myoepithelial carcinoma

- Cellular to hypercellular aspirates
- Single cells and large tissue fragments with crowding and overlapping consisting of neoplastic spindle cells typically predominate; however, epithelioid, plasmacytoid/hyaline, and /or clear cells also may be present
- Nuclei possess coarse chromatin with conspicuous nucleoli
- Mild-to-moderate cytological atypia
- Mitotic figures are unusual but may be present
- Stromal elements may be present in the background

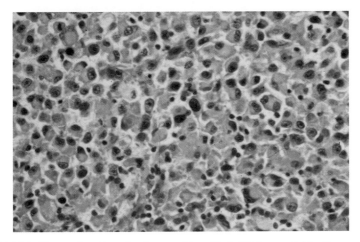

FIGURE 13.6. Sheets of moderately pleomorphic epithelioid/plasmacytoid cells, coarse chromatin, and variably distinct nucleoli are present with occasional binucleate cells. Sparse collagen bundles may be present. (Cell block, hematoxylin and eosin stain 100×). Courtesy of S. Kini, M.D., Henry Ford Hospital, Detroit, Michigan. NOTE: The diagnosis of malignancy hinges on histologic confirmation of infiltration.

Histologically, malignant myoepithelioma presents an infiltrative growth pattern, aiding in its diagnosis and is regarded as the minimum requirement for establishing the diagnosis of myoepithelial carcinoma. This feature cannot be assessed cytomorphologically and requires histological correlation. Two growth patterns may be observed in this entity, a multinodular growth pattern or the less common architectural variant in which large sheets and intervening hyaline or myxoid stroma predominate (Figure 13.6). Metachromatic stroma intermixed with neoplastic cells may be visualized histologically, regardless of the cellular subtype composition. Occasionally, perineural invasion and rarely dedifferentiation have been described.

13.3.3 Differential Diagnoses

Benign mixed tumors, particularly in cases with conspicuous stromal components resulting in a biphasic pattern and relatively little cytological atypia enter into the differential diagnosis. Further confounding this differential is consideration to carcinoma ex pleomorphic adenoma in which the malignant myoepithelial component in fact is associated with a preexisting pleomorphic adenoma. Similarly, the distinction of malignant myoepithelioma from benign myoepithelioma or the former developing in the latter may require a high index of suspicion based on clinical information and, ultimately, histologic confirmation. The differential diagnosis and clues to make the distinctions are summarized in Table 13.4.

TABLE 13.4. Differential diagnosis of myoepithelial carcinoma

	Clues to make the distinction
Pleomorphic adenoma	Two populations of cells — epithelial and myoepithelial cells
	Typically little to mild cytological atypia
Oncocytic tumors	Granular cytoplasmic features present
	Lack stromal elements
	Central nuclei
Malignant melanoma	Immunoprofiles as malignant melanoma (S-100, HMB-45, and Melan-A positive)
Spindle cell tumors	Appropriate spindle cell immunoprofile

Plasmacytoid cells in a myoepithelial carcinoma require distinction from oncocytic tumors. Careful attention to the nature of the granular cytoplasm of oncocytic neoplasms with centrally positioned nuclei contrast the non-granular cytoplasm of plasmacytoid myoepithelial cells that possess characteristic eccentric nuclei and, in some cases, hyperchromatic and atypical nuclei. The presence of neoplastic spindle cells also aids in this distinction, as these cells should be lacking oncocytic neoplasms. Malignant amelanotic melanoma, a notorious mimic of many neoplasms, possesses many overlapping features with malignant myoepithelioma including loosely cohesive spindle, plasmacytoid, or polygonal cells with prominent nucleoli, binucleation, and even rarely, intranuclear pseudoinclusions. Benign and malignant mesenchymal neoplasms, as mentioned in the previous discussion (see myoepithelioma), are differential diagnostic considerations in examples predominantly comprising spindle cells.

Ancillary studies, particularly immunohistochemistry, may be helpful in making the distinction. Myoepithelial cell differentiation is supported by immunoreactivity with cytokeratin, S-100, SMA, GFAP, and calponin. Malignant melanoma, also positive with S-100 protein, is supported further by immunoreactivity with human melanoma black (HMB)-45 and melan-A.

13.3.4 Treatment and Prognosis

Complete surgical excision in some cases is accompanied by lymph node dissection. The role of radiation therapy and chemotherapy may be contemplated. The presence of malignancy confined to pleomorphic adenomas or of benign myoepithelial tumors without capsular violation may influence the role of such additional therapy. Malignant myoepitheliomas are prone to recurrences and to locally aggressive behavior. Those that develop de novo behave no differently than those developing in association with preexisting benign salivary gland tumors, and with roughly equal probability, patients either die of disease, have several recurrences, or live free of disease.

13.4 EPITHELIAL-MYOEPITHELIAL (INTERCALATED DUCT) CARCINOMA

13.4.1 Clinical Features

The uncommon ($<1\%$ of salivary gland neoplasms) epithelial-myoepithelial carcinoma is a malignant neoplasm, with varying patterns of biological behavior. However, it generally is considered a low-grade carcinoma. Most occur in the parotid gland. There is a female preponderance (2:1) and a broad age range, with an average age of 62 years, a somewhat older age group than its benign counterpart. Approximately 40% may recur, and 14% metastasize, usually to cervical lymph nodes, liver, lung, or kidney.

13.4.2 Cytological Features and Histological Correlate

The tumor typically presents a cellular aspirate comprising three-dimensional clusters defined by a dual cell population, epithelial cells, and myoepithelial cells. Cellular aggregates are defined by centrally located, relatively smaller ductal epithelial cells with scant cytoplasm (Figure 13.7) often surrounded by peripherally positioned larger clear myoepithelial cells with moderately abundant glycogen-containing cytoplasm, vesicular nuclei, small/indistinct nucleoli, and sometimes mild-to-moderate cytological atypia; myoepithelial cells otherwise may be present as naked bipolar nuclei in the background. Hyaline material may be associated with these aggregates, a feature simulating hyaline globules reminiscent of adenoid cystic carcinoma (Figure 13.8). This entity may provoke a false-negative diagnosis, a challenge especially difficult when the tumor is cystic, a rare clinicopathologic presentation of such tumors. The key diagnostic features are summarized in Table 13.5.

Histologically, these tumors are well circumscribed, which may be, though are not necessarily, encapsulated, and present a proliferation of glandular elements separated by interposed fibroconnective tissue (Figure 13.9). The inner epithelial layer may be accentuated immunohistochemically by keratin markers and the outer myoepithelial layer by S-100, p63, colponin, SMA-HC, and SMA. Brisk mitotic activity, marked cytological atypia, hemorrhage, and necrosis are not likely present. The infiltrative architectural histologic pattern, a feature not discernible cytomorphologically, is paramount to an appropriate diagnosis (Figure 13.9).

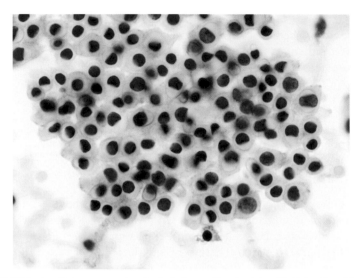

FIGURE 13.7. A cellular aggregate of relatively smaller ductal epithelial cells with scant to moderate cytoplasm and central round to slightly ovoid nuclei with evenly distributed chromatin. (Papanicolaou stain 400×). Courtesy of R.M. DeMay, M.D., University of Chicago Medical Center, Chicago, Illinois.

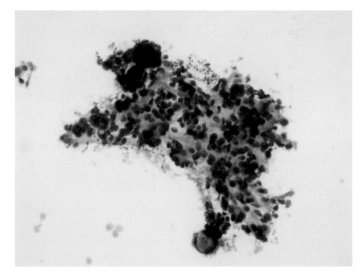

FIGURE 13.8. A sheet of epithelial-myoepithelial cells is present. Ductal epithelium line tubules surrounded by myoepithelial cells. Cell borders are somewhat indistinct. The cytoplasm is variable, and naked nuclei are also evident. Hyaline material may be associated with epithelial-myoepithelial aggregates, similar to hyaline globules reminiscent of adenoid cystic carcinoma. (Papanicolaou stain 640×). Courtesy of S. Kini, M.D., Henry Ford Hospital, Detroit, Michigan.

TABLE 13.5. Key diagnostic features of epithelial-myoepithelial carcinoma

- Cellular to hypercellular aspirates
- Three-dimensional clusters of cells presenting a dimorphic population: epithelial and myoepithelial cells
- Bipolar bare myoepithelial nuclei may be present in background
- Vesicular nuclei with small/indistinct nucleoli
- Cytological atypia varies from mild-marked
- Acellular material reminiscent of adenoid cystic basement membrane-type material often present
- Occasionally, increased mitotic figures present

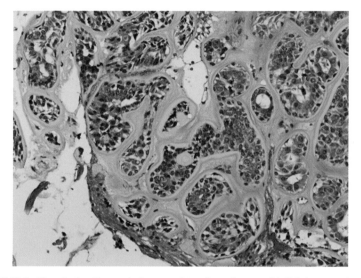

FIGURE 13.9. The dual cell population consists of an inner epithelial layer and an outer myoepithelial layer with varying degrees of cytologic atypia. (Cell block, hematoxylin and eosin stain 100×). Courtesy of R.M. DeMay, M.D., University of Chicago Medical Center, Chicago, Illinois. NOTE: Infiltration (not discernible cytologically), when observed in an excision specimen, cinches the diagnosis.

13.4.3 Differential Diagnoses

Differential diagnostic considerations of epithelial-myoepithelial carcinoma include pleomorphic adenoma and well-differentiated adenocarcinoma, both of which have similar cytomorphologic features. The histologic infiltrative nature of epithelial-myoepithelial carcinoma (not discernible cytomorphologically) may aid in the distinction of this entity from others.

TABLE 13.6. Differential diagnosis of epithelial-myoepithelial carcinoma	
	Clues to make the distinction
Pleomorphic adenoma	Dual cell population though epithelial cell population usually predominates Well-circumscribed
Well-differentiated adenocarcinoma	Dual cell population not characteristic
Adenoid cystic carcinoma	Small basaloid cells predominate with less conspicuous myoepithelial cell population Perineural infiltration (clinically, pain)

Dual cell populations may be observed in both pleomorphic adenoma and epithelial-myoepithelial carcinoma. Adenoid cystic carcinoma, a morphologic differential diagnostic consideration, typically comprises a predominant population of small, uniform, basaloid cells and a relatively less conspicuous population of myoepithelial cells. Characteristic metachromatic basement membrane-like material is present in spaces defined by the epithelial cell population. The differential diagnosis and clues to make the distinction are summarized in Table 13.6. Clinically, adenoid cystic carcinoma is associated with pain, correlating with perineural infiltration histologically, a feature not typically observed histologically in epithelial-myoepithelial carcinoma. Ultimately, distinction from adenoid cystic carcinoma, basal cell tumors, myoepithelial carcinoma, mucoepidermoid carcinoma, acinic cell carcinoma, polymorphous low-grade adenocarcinoma, or metastatic carcinomas consisting of clear cells (renal cell and others) may require clinical, gross, histologic, and immunohistochemical correlation (see previous discussions).

13.4.4 Treatment and Prognosis

Surgical excision with meticulously free margins is the mainstay treatment for this entity, which, depending on its location, may not always be feasible. The role of additional therapeutic intervention is not entirely clear, but as in the case of malignant myoepithelioma, may be considered depending on its histologic features. Size, rapid tumor growth, completeness of surgical excision, and marked cytological atypia are poor prognostic factors. The rarity of this tumor precludes definitive prognostic speculation.

Table 13.7 presents differential diagnostic features of myoepithelial tumors in general.

TABLE 13.7. Differential diagnosis of myoepithelial tumors

Myoepithelioma	Malignant myoepithelioma	Epithelial-myoepithelial carcinoma
Single cells and loosely cohesive groups of one or more cell types (spindle, epithelioid, clear, and plasmacytoid/hyaline)	Single cells and loosely cohesive tissue fragments of one or more cell types (spindle, epithelioid, clear, and plasmacytoid/hyaline)	Cellular to hypercellular aspirate that consists of a dual cell population
Honeycomb sheets of epithelial cells lacking	Three-dimensional groups with nuclear crowding and overlapping	Three-dimensional clusters defined by dual cell population Centrally located smaller epithelial cells surrounded by myoepithelial cells
Fine chromatin, inconspicuous, small nucleoli	Coarse chromatin with prominent nucleoli	Vesicular nuclei with small/indistinct nucleoli
Minimal cytological atypia with the exception of plasmacytoid variant, which may present pleomorphic nuclei	Variable cytological atypia (may be marked atypia), pleomorphism, and possible necrosis	Marked atypia, brisk mitoses, hemorrhage, and necrosis typically absent
No stromal elements	Neoplastic cells and metachromatic stromal fragments	Hyaline stromal material surrounds cellular aggregates
Few if any mitoses	Bi-, multinucleation, and occasional mitoses	Mitotic activity typically inconspicuous
	May develop de novo, or in preexisting pleomorphic adenoma (carcinoma ex pleomorphic adenoma) or myoepithelioma	
Lack of infiltrative pattern histologically	Infiltrative growth pattern histologically p53 staining, ≥10% Ki-67 staining may support malignant diagnostic interpretation	Infiltrative growth pattern histologically

RECOMMENDED READINGS

Barnes L, Eveson JW, Reichart P, Sidransky D, editors. World Health Organization Classification of Tumours. Pathology & Genetics of Head and Neck Tumours. Lyon (France): IARC Press; 2005.

Bombi JA, Alos L, Rey MJ, Mallofre C, Cuchi A, Trasserra J, Cardsa A. Myoepithelial carcinoma arising in a benign myoepithelioma: immunohistochemical, ultrastructural, and flow-cytometrical study. Ultrastruct Pathol 1996;20: 145–154.

Chieng DC, Paulino AF. Cytology of myoepithelial carcinoma of the salivary gland: a study of four cases. Cancer (Cancer Cytopathol) 2002;96:32–36.

Chow LT, Chow WH, Lee JC. Monomorphic epithelioid variant of malignant myoepithelioma of the parotid gland: cytologic features in fine needle aspiration (FNA). Cytopathology 1996;7:279–287.

Daneshbod Y, Daneshbod K, Khademi B. Diagnostic difficulties in the interpretation of fine needle aspirate samples in salivary lesions: diagnostic pitfalls revisited. Acta Cytol 2009;53:53–70.

DeMay R. Art & Science of Cytopathology, Aspiration Cytology. Chicago (IL): ASCP Press; 1996.

DiPalma S, Alasio L, Pilotti S. Fine needle aspiration (FNA) appearances of malignant myoepithelioma of the parotid gland. Cytopathology 1996;7:357–365.

Ellis G, Auclair P, Gnepp D. Surgical Pathology of Salivary Glands. Philadelphia, PA: Saunders; 1991.

Hata M, Tokuuye K, Shioyama Y, Nomoto S, Inadome Y, Fukumitsu N, Nakayama H, Sugahara S, Ohara K, Noguchi M, Akine Y. Malignant Myoepithelioma in the maxillary sinus: case report and review of the literature. Anticancer Res 2009;29:497–501.

Isogai R, Kawada A, Ueno K, Aragane Y, Tezuka T. Myoepithelioma possibly originating from the accessory parotid gland. Dermatology 2004;208:74–78.

Nagao T, Sugano I, Ishida Y, Taima Y, Matsuzaki O, Konno A, Kondo Y, Nagao K. Salivary gland malignant myoepithelioma: a clinicopathologic and immunohistochemical study of ten cases. Cancer 1998;83:1292–1299.

Ogawa I, Nishida t, Miyauchi M, Sato S, Takata T. Dedifferentiated malignant myoepithelioma of the parotid gland. Pathol Int 2003;53:704–709.

Rosai J. Rosai and Ackerman's Surgical Pathology, Volume 1. Philadelphia (PA): Mosby; 2004.

Savera AT, Sloman A, Huvos AG, Klimstra DS. Myoepithelial carcinoma of the salivary glands: a clinicopathologic study of 25 patients. Am J Surg Pathol 2000;24:761–774.

Seifert G. Histological typing of salivary gland tumors. In: Sobin LH, editor. World Health Organization International Histological Classification of Tumours. Berlin (Germany): Springer-Verlag; 1991.

Stewart CJ, MacKenzie K, McGarry GW, Mowat A. Fine-needle aspiration cytology of salivary gland: a review of 341 cases. Diagn Cytopathol 2000;22:139–146.

Stromeyer FW, Haggitt RC, Nelson JF, Hardman JM. Myoepithelioma of minor salivary gland origin. Light and electron microscopical study. Arch Pathol Lab Med 1975;99:242–245.

Torlakovic E, Ames ED, Manivel JC, Stanley MW. Benign and malignant neoplasms of myoepithelial cells: cytologic findings. Diagn Cytopathol 1993;9:655–660.

CHAPTER 14

POLYMORPHOUS LOW-GRADE CARCINOMA

JERZY KLIJANIENKO, MD, PHD, MIAC and MOUSA A. AL-ABBADI, MD, FIAC

14.1 INTRODUCTION

Polymorphous low-grade adenocarcinoma is a relatively recently described low-grade carcinoma that develops predominantly from minor salivary glands, particularly from the palate. It is characterized by cytologic uniformity and histologic diversity with infiltration to surrounding structures. It represents approximately 5% of all salivary glands tumors.

14.2 CLINICAL FEATURES

This tumor affects adults, mainly in the sixth decade, with clear female predominance. Tumor origin is almost limited to the oral cavity, palate, and upper lips. Patients present with a painless yellow, firm, mass that feels usually well circumscribed but nonencapsulated. A preexcision fine needle aspiration is not common, and in most cases, the diagnosis is made on histological examination.

14.3 CYTOLOGICAL FEATURES AND HISTOLOGICAL CORRELATES

Cytologically, smears are rich and comprise of both cellular and connective tissue components. Cells are round, observed in clusters, and occasionally

Salivary Gland Cytology: A Color Atlas, Edited by Mousa A. Al-Abbadi
Copyright © 2011 Wiley-Blackwell

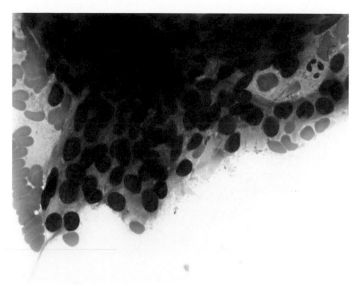

FIGURE 14.1. High power smears with cellular clusters of cuboidal-round cells with regular and clarified nuclei and slightly ample agranular cytoplasm. The cells and nuclei are uniform and bland (May–Grünwald–Giemsa [MGG], 400×).

isolated (Figure 14.1). The cytoplasm is usually stripped and eosinophilic. The nuclei are vescicular and clarified with delicate chromatin and minimal pleomorphism. Mitotic figures are absent. The aspirated associated stroma consists of hyaline globules similar to those of adenoid cystic carcinoma (Figures 14.2 and 14.3). They appear in eosinophilic/magenta red cores that may branch in bands with the associated epithelial papillary structures (Figure 14.3). Table 14.1 summarizes the key cytologic features.

A large variety of histological features is noted in polymorphous low-grade adenocarcinoma, hence the name polymorphous. The growth patterns include solid islands (Figure 14.4); tubular, trabecular, cribriform nests; cystic; and papillary projections. Perineural and bone invasions are often present. Cells are small, cuboidal, and/or columnar and bland. Nuclei are vesicular and mitoses are rare (Figure 14.4).

14.4 THE MAJOR CYTOLOGICAL DIFFERENTIAL DIAGNOSIS AND CLUES TO MAKE THE DISTINCTION

The presence of hyaline globules creates a differential diagnosis with adenoid cystic carcinoma, pleomorphic adenoma, and epi-myoepithelial carcinoma. In adenoid cystic carcinoma, the cells are basaloid with smaller nuclei and scant

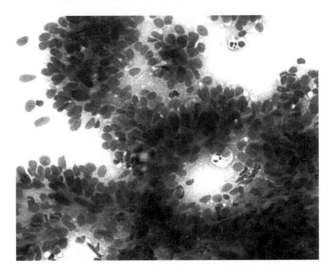

FIGURE 14.2. Tubular and papillary structures with magenta hyaline globules in branching bands surrounded by the associated epithelial structures (MGG, 200×).

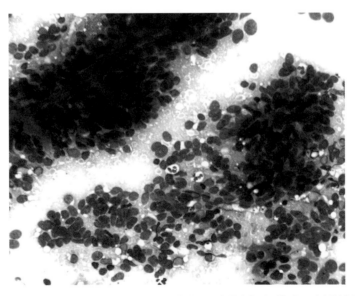

FIGURE 14.3. Papillary structures, hyaline globules, and slightly clarified nuclei (MGG, 200×).

cytoplasm. The nuclear chromatin is coarse and dark, there is more nuclear pleomorphism, and mitoses are usually observed. In contrast to pleomorphic adenoma, the chondromyxoid stroma and the abundant plasmacytoid myoepithelial cells are absent in polymorphous low-grade adenocarcinoma.

TABLE 14.1. Key cytologic features of polymorphous low grade adenocarcinoma

- Round/cuboidal or columnar cells in papillary clusters
- Clarified and isomorphic nuclei with delicate vesicular chromatin
- No mitoses
- Hyaline globules in cores and branching bands with associated papillae
- Minor salivary glands (especially palate)

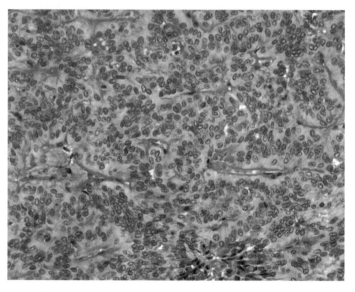

FIGURE 14.4. The solid areas, one of many fields of diverse histologic features of polymorphous low-grade adenocarcinoma, which shows clear nuclei surrounding vascular cores. Other fields show clear infiltration by these bland-appearing cells (hematoxylin and eosin, 200×).

Epi-myoepithelial carcinoma, when well differentiated, shows the presence of a double population of darker (ductal) and clear (myoepithelial) cells. Table 14.2 summarizes the differential diagnosis.

14.5 TREATMENT OF CHOICE AND PROGNOSIS

Complete surgical removal is the only therapeutic modality. Despite local aggressiveness, the prognosis is excellent and distant metastasis is exceptional.

TABLE 14.2. Major differential diagnoses of polymorphous low-grade adenocarcinoma

	Clues to make the distinction
Adenoid cystic carcinoma	The presence of tubular structures and finger-like structures are characteristic for adenoid cystic carcinoma. However, adenoid cystic carcinoma mainly consists of basaloid cells with mitoses. Nuclei are irregular, whereas the nuclei in polymorphous low-grade adenocarcinoma are clarified and isomorphic. In addition, in contrast to polymorphous low-grade adenocarcinoma, adenoid cystic carcinoma is rare in the palate.
Pleomorphic adenoma	The chondromyxoid stroma and plasmacytoid myoepithelial cells are absent in polymorphous low-grade adenocarcinoma.
Epi-myoepithelial carcinoma	May be difficult to differentiate. Epi-myoepithelial carcinoma frequently shows a bimodal cell population of ductal cells and clarified, myoepithelial cells. In addition, polymorphous low-grade adenocarcinoma develops in the minor salivary glands.

RECOMMENDED READINGS

Bastakis JG, Pinkston GR, Luna MA, Byers RM, Sciubba JJ, Tillery GW. Adenocarcinoma of the oral cavity: a clinicopathologic study of terminal duct carcinoma. J Laryngol Otol 1983;97:825–835.

Castle JT, Thompson LD, Frommelt RA, Wenig BM, Kessler HP. Polymorphous low grade adenocarcinoma: a clinicopathologic study of 164 cases. Cancer 1999;86;207–219.

Klijanienko J, Vielh P. Salivary carcinomas with papillae: cytology and histology analysis of polymorphous low-grade adenocarcinoma and papillary cystadenocarcinoma. Diagn Cytopathol 1998;19:244–249.

Klijanienko J, Vielh P, Batsakis JD, el-Naggar AK, Jelen M, Piekarski JD. Salivary gland tumours. In: Orell SR, editor. Monographs in Clinical Cytology. Volume 15. Basel (Switzerland): Karger; 2000. p III–XII, 1–138.

McHugh JB, Visscher DW, Barnes EL. Update on selected salivary gland neoplasms. Arch Pathol Lab Med 2010;133:1763–1774.

Waldron CA, el Mofty SK, Gnepp DR. Tumors of the intraoral minor salivary glands: a demographic and histologic study of 426 cases. Oral Surg Oral Med Oral Pathol 1988;66:323–333.

CHAPTER 15

SALIVARY DUCT CARCINOMA

JERZY KLIJANIENKO, MD, PHD, MIAC and MOUSA A. AL-ABBADI, MD, FIAC

15.1 INTRODUCTION

Salivary glands and breast tissue are of the same embryological origin and are both skin adnexa. Primary salivary duct carcinoma is a high-grade malignancy related morphologically to mammary ductal adenocarcinoma, which is why it is important to exclude the presence of primary mammary carcinoma at the time of diagnosis. This entity represents approximately 3% of all salivary gland tumors. For a long period of time, salivary duct carcinoma was considered under the broader category of "salivary adenocarcinoma not otherwise specified." However, currently all agree that it represents a specific unique entity. Occasionally, salivary duct carcinoma may develop in pleomorphic adenoma. Moreover, a "low-grade variant" of salivary duct carcinoma has been described. It is also worthwhile to mention that similar tumors have been reported in lacrimal glands.

15.2 CLINICAL FEATURES

This carcinoma occurs in the parotid gland with male predominance in the sixth and sevenths decade of life. Because of its high-grade nature, patients present with a recently enlarging, painful, and fixed parotid mass. Cervical lymph node metastases and distant metastases are frequently present at the time of diagnosis.

15.3 CYTOLOGICAL FEATURES AND HISTOLOGICAL CORRELATE

Cytologically, salivary duct carcinoma is similar to high-grade ductal mammary carcinoma. Smears are richly cellular with obviously malignant cells with an abundant background of necrosis. Cells are frequently clustered, but single malignant cells are also observed. The cells are pleomorphic and have well-preserved cytoplasm. Occasionally, tubular, glandular, and papillary formations are observed. Nuclei are large and contain prominent nucleoli. Cellular and nuclear atypia is prominent, and numerous mitotic figures are present. The background contains extensive necrosis, apoptotic debris, macrophages, and numerous leukocytes are observed. Cells around necrotic areas show an oncocytic cytopalsmic change with vacuolization (Figures 15.1–15.4). Table 15.1 summarizes the key diagnostic cytological features of salivary duct carcinoma.

Histologically, salivary duct carcinoma resembles high-grade mammary comedocarcinoma. Cells are in sheaths, cords, and clusters. Glandular differentiation is well appreciated with cribriforming and occasional papillary projections into cystic spaces. However, the hallmark is central necrosis of solid areas (Figure 15.5).

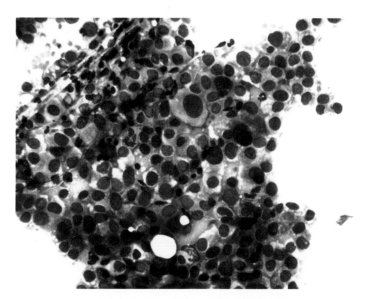

FIGURE 15.1. Marked cellular and nuclear atypia (May–Grünwald–Giemsa [MGG], 200×).

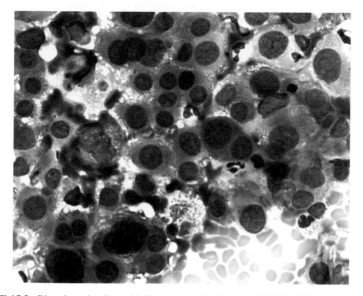

FIGURE 15.2. Binucleated cells and inflammatory background (MGG, 400×).

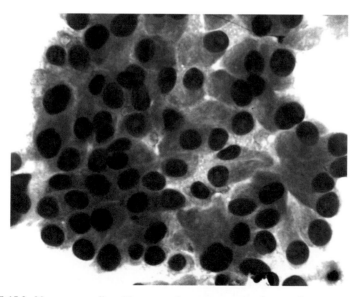

FIGURE 15.3. Numerous cells with oncocytic pattern around necrotic areas are shown (MGG, 200×).

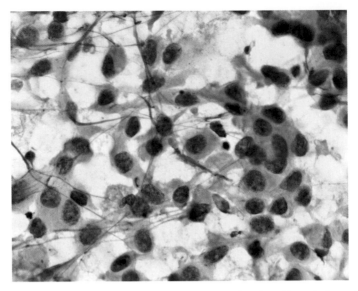

FIGURE 15.4. Necrotic and inflammatory background is abundant (Papanicolaou, 400×).

TABLE 15.1. Key cytologic features of salivary duct carcinoma
• Cellular smears
• Significant cellular and nuclear atypia and pleomorphism
• Frequent mitotic figures
• Background dirty necrosis with numerous neutrophils
• Occasional atypical oncocytic or microvacuolated cells

15.4 MAJOR CYTOLOGICAL DIFFERENTIAL DIAGNOSIS AND CLUES TO MAKE THE DISTINCTION

Although it is sometimes difficult to separate different high-grade carcinomas of the salivary gland merely on cytological grounds, for clinical purposes, the distinction may not be needed because all carcinomas require aggressive radical surgery. The main differential diagnosis of salivary duct carcinoma is high-grade mucoepidermoid carcinoma, oncocytic carcinoma, and metastatic carcinoma. In high-grade mucoepidermoid carcinoma smears, squamoid and squamous cell carcinoma cells are usually observed in addition to mucinous cells and mucoid background. These cells are rarely observed in salivary duct carcinoma. Necrosis can be present in both entities; therefore, this feature is not helpful.

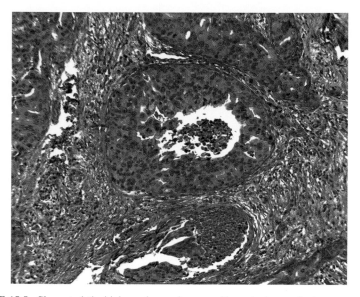

FIGURE 15.5. Characteristic high-grade carcinoma with central comedo-type necrosis and stromal infiltration (hematoxylin and eosin, 200×).

Salivary duct carcinomas rich in oncocytic cells should be differentiated from salivary malignant oncocytoma or metastatic Hurthle cell carcinoma of the thyroid. The distinction is not always possible solely on cytomorphological grounds. Necrosis is usually scant in oncocytic carcinoma, and the cytoplasm is more abundant and granular than that of salivary duct carcinoma. In addition, the nuclear atypia is more pronounced, and the chromatin is more coarse in oncocytic carcinoma. Hurthle cell carcinoma may require thyroid evaluation in the absence of history and additional immunohistochemical stains on cell block material (Table 15.2).

15.5 TREATMENT OF CHOICE AND PROGNOSIS

This tumor is very aggressive and harbors a poor prognosis. Treatment is based on surgery, radiotherapy, and chemotherapy. Several studies were undertaken for therapeutic purposes using N-Myc, estrogen, and progesterone receptors. However, one third of the patients develop local recurrence and almost half develop distant metastasis. Metastasis involves the lung, bone, liver, brain, and skin.

TABLE 15.2. Major differential diagnoses of salivary duct carcinoma	
	Clues to make the distinction
High-grade mucoepidermoid carcinoma	The presence of squamoid and mucus-secreting cells are strongly in favor of high-grade mucoepidermoid carcinoma.
Malignant oncocytoma	The differential diagnosis may be difficult. Abundant granular cytoplasm, nuclear atypia, and coarse chromatin usually are observed in oncocytic carcinoma. Necrosis is usually absent or scant in malignant oncocytoma.
Metastatic hurthle cell carcinoma	In the absence of history, the distinction is difficult. Immunohistochemical stains for thyroglobulin and thyroglobulin transcription factor-1 (TTF-1) are usually positive in Hurthle cell carcinoma of thyroid.

RECOMMENDED READINGS

Barnes L, Rao U, Krause J, Contis L, Schwartz A. Salivary duct carcinoma. Part I. A clinicopathologic evaluation and DNA image analysis of 13 cases with review of the literature. Oral Surg Oral Med Oral Path 1994;78:74–80.

Klijanienko J, Vielh P. Cytologic characteristics and histomorphologic correlations of 21 salivary duct carcinomas. Diagn Cytopathol 1998;19:333–337.

Klijanienko J, Vielh P, Batsakis JD, el-Naggar AK, Jelen M, Piekarski JD. Salivary gland tumors. In: Orell SR, editor. Monographs in Clinical Cytology. Volume 15. Basel, Switzerland: Karger; 2000. p III–XII, 1–138.

CHAPTER 16

SALIVARY GLAND LYMPHOMAS

MOHAMMAD ABUEL-HAIJA, MD
MAGDALENA CZADER, MD, PHD

16.1 INTRODUCTION

Primary lymphomas of salivary glands are rare and represent less than 2% of primary salivary gland neoplasms. Similar to lymph nodes, most salivary gland lymphomas are derived from mature B cells. Marginal zone lymphoma of mucosa-associated lymphoid tissue is the most common salivary gland lymphoma and frequently develops in association with reactive lymphoid proliferations in autoimmune conditions. Less common are follicular lymphoma and diffuse large B-cell lymphoma. The latter can be primary or develop as a transformation of low-grade lymphoid neoplasm. Parotid and submandibular glands are the predominant sites of involvement. Minor salivary gland lymphomas are less common.

Because of the overlap in cytologic features, the definitive diagnosis and subclassification of salivary gland lymphoma on cytology alone is frequently challenging. Cytologic evaluation of fine needle aspiration (FNA) commonly is accompanied by immunophenotyping by flow cytometry or immunohistochemistry of a cell block.

16.2 HODGKIN LYMPHOMA

16.2.1 Introduction

Hodgkin lymphoma, formerly known as Hodgkin disease, has been described first by Thomas Hodgkin in 1832. The controversy over the origin of this

Salivary Gland Cytology: A Color Atlas, Edited by Mousa A. Al-Abbadi
Copyright © 2011 Wiley-Blackwell

lymphoma lasted more than a century and led to the original designation as Hodgkin disease or lymphogranulomatosis. With the demonstration of the B-cell origin of this neoplasm, the term Hodgkin lymphoma has been introduced. The World Health Organization (WHO) classification of lymphoid and hematopoietic tumors divides Hodgkin lymphoma into two categories—nodular lymphocyte-predominant Hodgkin lymphoma and classical Hodgkin lymphoma (cHL). Nodular lymphocyte-predominant Hodgkin lymphoma consists of lymphocytic/histiocytic or "popcorn" cells scattered within nodules of reactive lymphocytes. It rarely involves extranodal sites and thus is not discussed in this chapter in detail. cHL is characterized by the presence of Reed-Sternberg (RS) cells in a rich reactive inflammatory background. The cHL is observed most frequently in lymph nodes and other lymphoid organs such as the spleen and liver. It occasionally presents in extranodal sites, especially in immunodeficient individuals. The cHL is divided into the following histologic subtypes: nodular sclerosis, mixed cellularity, lymphocyte-rich, and lymphocyte-depleted.

16.2.2 Clinical Features

Classical Hodgkin lymphoma presents most frequently in lymph nodes and can involve related lymphoid organs such as the spleen and liver. Cervical lymphadenoapthy is most common followed by mediastinal, axillary, or paraaortic lymph node involvement. Bone marrow is involved in 5% of cases. Primary extranodal site cHL is rare in immunocompetent individuals and is more frequent in the immunodeficient population. Rare reports of salivary gland involvement have been published in the literature. B symptoms including fever, weight loss, and night sweats are common in cHL.

16.2.3 Cytologic Features with Histologic Correlates

Fine needle aspirations of cHL can be variably cellular depending on the histologic subtype of the lesion. The lymphocyte-rich and mixed cellularity types usually yield a richly cellular sample with most cells being small lymphocytes admixed with rare neoplastic cells. The nodular sclerosis cHL may be difficult to aspirate because of extensive fibrosis. The aspirate can contain fibroblasts and metachromatic fibrillar material derived from collagenous bands characteristic of nodular sclerosis cHL.

Regardless of the histologic subtype, the pathognomonic findings are the presence of RS cells in a reactive inflammatory background comprising small lymphocytes, plasma cells, histiocytes, and eosinophils (Figure 16.1a and b, Table 16.1). Granulomatous reaction and necrotic foci can be present. The RS cells are required for the diagnosis and are present in each histologic subtype of cHL. The typical RS cell is a large lymphoid cell, of an average size of 40–70 μm, with a bilobed nucleus or two nuclei with prominent centrally

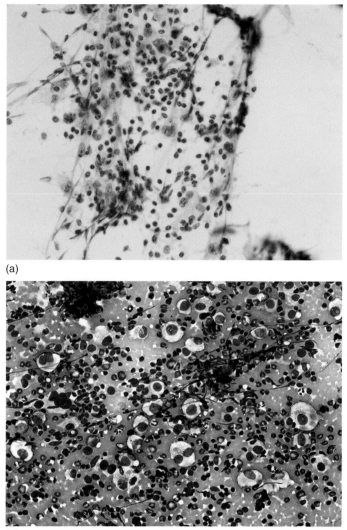

(a)

(b)

FIGURE 16.1. (*Continued*)

located inclusion-like nucleolus and abundant cytoplasm (Figure 16.1c). The appearance of the nuclei sometimes is compared with the image of an owl's eyes. In Papanicolaou stain, the characteristic nucleoli of RS cells stain bright red. The cytoplasm is abundant and stains usually blue-green in Papanicolaou and basophilic in Diff-Quik stain. The variants of RS cells such as mononuclear Hodgkin cells, lacunar cells, and mummified cells are observed frequently; however, they are not sufficient for the diagnosis of

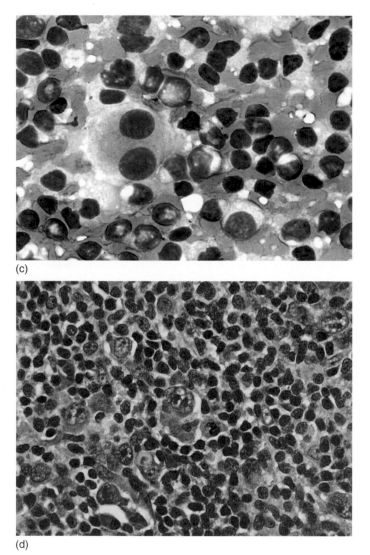

(c)

(d)

FIGURE 16.1. Classical Hodgkin lymphoma. (**a**) FNA of nodular sclerosis cHL showing cohesive aggregates including small lymphocytes, histiocytes, fibroblasts granulocytes, and scattered RS and Hodgkin cells (Papanicolaou, 500×). (**b**) Occasionally, aspirates of cHL show numerous RS and Hodgkin cells. In such cases, differential diagnosis includes DLBCL and nonlymphoid neoplasms (Diff-Quik, 600×). (**c**) In Diff-Quik stain, classic RS cells have blue cytoplasm and distinct inclusion-like nucleoli (1000×). (**d**) Classical RS cells (center) in a histologic section from cHL (hematoxylin and eosin, 1000×).

cHL (Figure 16.1d). Mononuclear Hodgkin cells are large lymphoid cells with a single nucleus, distinct nucleolus, and abundant cytoplasm. Lacunar cells are appreciated best in the histologic sections (needle biopsies or cell blocks). They may be mononuclear with oval or multilobated nuclei, or multinucleated, and

TABLE 16.1. Key diagnostic features of salivary gland lymphomas

Lymphoma subtype	Key diagnostic features
Classical Hodgkin lymphoma	Reed-Sternberg cells in a rich background of small lymphocytes, plasma cells, histiocytes, and eosinophils
Extranodal marginal zone lymphoma of mucosa-associated lymphoid tissue	Noncohesive polymorphous lymphoid population encompassing predominantly small and medium-sized lymphocytes, with dense chromatin, and oval-to-irregular nuclei. Plasma cells and large lymphoid cells are present
Follicular lymphoma	Low-grade (histologic grade 1–2): population of small- to medium-sized centrocytes with cleaved nuclei (can be angular or indented) with noticeable, however, infrequent centroblasts High-grade (histologic grade 3): predominance of centroblasts (large lymphoid cells with oval nuclei and multiple peripheral nucleoli) cytologically indistinguishable from DLBCL
Diffuse large B-cell lymphoma	Cellular FNA smear showing numerous noncohesive large lymphoid cells, which can demonstrate nuclear pleomorphism, abundant cytoplasm and prominent nucleoli
Plasma cell neoplasm	Noncohesive cells with eccentric nuclei, distinct nucleoli, clock-face chromatin, and perinuclear hof. Intranuclear (Dutcher) and intracytopalsmic (Russel) inclusions may be present. Binucleated forms can be observed

show cytoplasm retraction in formalin fixed tissue. Mummified cells have pyknotic nuclei and condensed cytoplasm. Nucleoli are difficult to appreciate. Because select non-Hodgkin lymphomas closely can resemble cHL cytologically, immunohistochemical stains, described in the following paragraphs, are required for a definitive diagnosis.

Histologic features of cHL are dependent on the subtype. Briefly, nodular sclerosis cHL, the most common type accounting for approximately 70% of cHL cases, shows broad collagen bands transsecting the lymph node and thickening of the nodal capsule. Lacunar cells frequently are present in this type of cHL. The background cellularity includes small lymphocytes, eosinophils, and histiocytes. In mixed cellularity cHL, fibrotic bands and capsular thickening are absent, and RS cells are scattered among the diffuse background proliferation of small lymphocytes, histiocytes, eosinophils, neutrophils, and plasma cells. Lymphocyte-rich type shows a vaguely nodular background of small lymphocytes with scattered RS cells. The RS cells and variants are most frequent in lymphocyte-depleted cHL, which is characterized by a paucity of a reactive background.

The demonstration of RS cells positive for CD30 and CD15 and negative for CD45 and T-cell markers is essential for the diagnosis. Immunohistochemical stain for the CD20 antigen can be weakly positive in a proportion of RS cells; however, at the time of primary diagnosis, staining is typically heterogeneous and not as intense as in cases of non-Hodgkin B-cell lymphomas. Relapsed cHL with strong CD20 immuno-reactivity has been reported. The cellular composition of background lymphoid cells is variable and dependent on the subtype of cHL. In most cases, CD4-positive T cells predominate. In lymphocyte-rich cHL, RS cells are embedded in remnants of mantle zones and follicles, comprising mainly B-cells; thus, immunophenotyping shows a more prominent B-cell background. Immunophenotype of RS cells is demonstrated best by immuno-histochemistry of a cell block.

16.2.4   Differential Diagnosis

Close attention is essential to both the cytology of neoplastic cells and to the reactive background. A host of other lymphoid malignancies and select reactive conditions closely can resemble cHL (Table 16.2). The most common reactive conditions, which cytologically can mimick cHL, are infectious mononucleosis and other reactive lymphoid proliferations containing immunoblasts, which occasionally resemble RS and Hodgkin cells. Reactive immunoblastic proliferations most commonly are associated with viral infections and autoimmune conditions. They typically show a continuum of cell cytology from small lymphocytes, through medium-sized lymphoid cells, and to large transformed lymphocytes. The latter may be bi- or multinucleated and feature large distinct nucleoli. In contrast, in cHL, one usually appreciates isolated RS and Hodgkin cells in an inflammatory background that may include small lymphoid cells, plasma cells, granulocytes, plasma cells, and histiocytes. The intermediate size lymphoid cells and cytologic continuum is not present. Granulomatous foci with epithelioid histiocytes also can be present in cases of cHL; thus, fine needle aspirations of any lesion with granulomatous inflammation have to be scrutinized closely for the presence of RS cells to exclude cHL.

The neoplasm most closely resembling cHL on cytologic examination is T cell/histiocyte-rich large B-cell lymphoma (THRLBCL), a subtype of diffuse large B-cell lymphoma (DLBCL). In this entity, rare neoplastic B cells are scattered in the reactive background comprising small lymphocytes with a variable admixture of histiocytes. Malignant cells can be pleomorphic and mimic RS and Hodgkin cells. However, T-cell/histiocyte-rich large B-cell

TABLE 16.2. Differential diagnosis of classical Hodgkin lymphoma	
Major differential diagnosis	Clues to make the distinction
Reactive conditions containing atypical immunoblasts resembling RS and Hodgkin cells frequently associated with viral infections	Reactive lymphoid proliferations most frequently show a continuum of lymphoid cell cytology from small- to medium-sized to large pleomorphic forms. On the contrary, cHL is characterized by RS cells and variant Hodgkin cells immersed in inflammatory background, no transitional forms, or cytologic continuum is observed
T cell/histiocyte-rich large B-cell lymphoma (THRLBCL), and other subtypes of DLBCL	If THRLBCL contain large pleomorphic cells, then it is cytologically indistinguishable from cHL. THRLBCL is rare at extranodal sites, and thus infrequently will be considered in the differential diagnosis. Other DLBCL subtypes usually have frequent large cells, which aid in the differentiation from cHL. In contrast to cHL, all DLBCL are positive for several B-cell markers such as CD20 and CD79a and the panhematopoietic antigen CD45 (LCA)
Anaplastic large cell lymphoma	ALCL can present with a rich inflammatory background, and these cases are challenging to distinguish from cHL unless IHC is performed to confirm T-cell/null immunophenotype and/or positivity for the ALK-1 antigen. The presence of numerous neoplastic cells and hallmark cells support the diagnosis of ALCL

ALCL = anaplastic large cell lymphoma; IHC = immunohistochemistry; LCA = leukocyte common antigen; THRLBCL = T cell/histiocyte-rich large B-cell lymphoma.

lymphoma rarely involves tissues outside of the lymphoid system or bone marrow and, based on the site of involvement, rarely will enter the differential diagnosis in lesions of salivary glands.

Typical diffuse large B-cell lymphoma more commonly involves salivary glands and in select cases can contain pleomorphic cells resembling RS and Hodgkin cells. In these cases, large cells predominate; thus, the main differential diagnosis will include lymphocyte-depleted or a syncytial variant of nodular sclerosis cHL. In such rare cases, immunohistochemical stains of cell block or flow cytometric immunophenotyping of fine needle aspirate are helpful in rendering a definitive diagnosis. Similarly, an immunophenotype is required for the differentiation between cHL and anaplastic large cell lymphoma, two entities shown to be misdiagnosed most frequently in nodal fine needle aspirates. Anaplastic large cell lymphoma, reported to rarely involve the parotid gland, consists of pleomorphic lymphoid cells with large nuclei, bi- or multinucleation, and abundant cytoplasm. A rich inflammatory background can be present. Wreath-like nuclei of neoplastic cells suggest anaplastic large cell lymphoma; however, final diagnosis requires immunohistochemical stains.

Rarely, other lymphoid malignancies, such as small lymphocytic lymphoma can contain RS-like cells, either at the time of original diagnosis or at the time of transformation (non-Hodgkin lymphoma as Richter transformation). These cases are rare and will require immunophenotyping to assess the nature of the background small lymphocytic proliferation adequately.

Finally, when numerous and clustering of RS and Hodgkin cells are encountered in FNA of a syncytial variant of nodular sclerosis cHL, a differential diagnosis includes poorly differentiated carcinoma, sarcoma, and melanoma.

16.2.5   Treatment and Prognosis

The cHL is treated with combination chemotherapy and/or radiation. The choice of treatment modality is based on the stage of the disease. More than 85% of patients are cured with this approach. Staging and laboratory features are used for prognostication. The best outcome occurs in patients with lymphocyte-rich and nodular sclerosis cHL, and the worst survival has been reported for the lymphocyte-depleted type.

16.3   EXTRANODAL MARGINAL ZONE LYMPHOMA OF MUCOSA-ASSOCIATED LYMPHOID TISSUE (MALT LYMPHOMA)

16.3.1   Introduction

Extranodal marginal zone lymphoma of mucosa-associated lymphoid tissue (MALT lymphoma) is the most common type of primary lymphoma in salivary glands. The original description of Mikulicz disease by Jan Mikulicz-Radecki in 1892 most likely represents the first description of salivary gland MALT lymphoma.

MALT lymphoma develops from postgerminal center memory B-cells, most frequently in patients with an autoimmune disease such as Sjogren syndrome, and is preceded by an acquisition of prominent mucosa-associated lymphoid tissue. The neoplastic population of MALT lymphoma is heterogeneous and includes small- and medium-sized lymphocytes, plasma cells, and occasional large lymphoid cells. The cytologic features overlap to a large extent with myoepithelial/lymphoepithelial sialadenitis (benign lymphoepithelial lesion), which makes cytologic diagnosis of MALT lymphoma one of the most challenging in salivary gland pathology.

16.3.2 Clinical Features

MALT lymphoma of salivary glands is the most frequent subtype of malignant lymphoma developing at this site. Parotid glands predominantly are involved. MALT lymphoma frequently presents with diffuse symmetric bilateral enlargement of salivary glands. Adults are affected most commonly, and there is a significant female predominance. Most patients have a prior history of autoimmune disease, predominantly Sjogren syndrome. This patient group have a 44-fold increased risk of developing lymphoma, which can be preceded by a benign lymphoepithelial lesion. The clinical course is usually indolent, and lymphoma remains confined to salivary glands. Rarely, patients develop disseminated disease and/or transformation to diffuse large B-cell lymphoma. Paraproteinemia may be present.

16.3.3 Cytologic Features with Histologic Correlates

MALT lymphoma consists of a population of small-to-intermediate-sized lymphocytes with abundant cytoplasm, irregular nuclear borders, and occasional nucleoli (monocytoid and centrocyte-like cells; Figure 16.2a and b, Table 16.1). The numbers of small lymphocytes, plasma cells, histiocytes, and large lymphoid cells vary from case to case. MALT lymphoma develops from postgerminal center memory B-cells; thus, in select cases, the plasmacytic differentiation can be significant and lead to the diagnosis of plasma cell neoplasm.

MALT lymphoma can efface the architecture of the salivary gland or involve only a portion of a gland. The proliferation is most commonly diffuse with distinct lymphoepithelial lesions representing infiltration of neoplastic lymphocytes into epithelium (Figure 16.2c). The lymphoepithelial lesions occur frequently in salivary glands; however, they are not required for the diagnosis. A characteristic feature, especially helpful when the neoplastic infiltrate is not prominent, is the presence of aggregates of monocytoid and centrocyte-like cells surrounding epimyoepithelial islands in histologic sections. The neoplastic population is heterogeneous and includes medium-sized lymphocytes, plasma cells, and scattered large lymphoid cells. Medium-sized marginal zone cells with irregular nuclei and relatively abundant cytoplasm predominate in most cases. Plasma cell differentiation can be prominent. In histologic sections, the differentiation between plasma cell neoplasm and MALT lymphoma with prominent plasmacytic differentiation is aided by immunophenotypic studies. The demonstration of a monoclonal population of B-lymphocytes and residual follicles favors the diagnosis of MALT lymphoma. Large lymphocytes can be frequent in

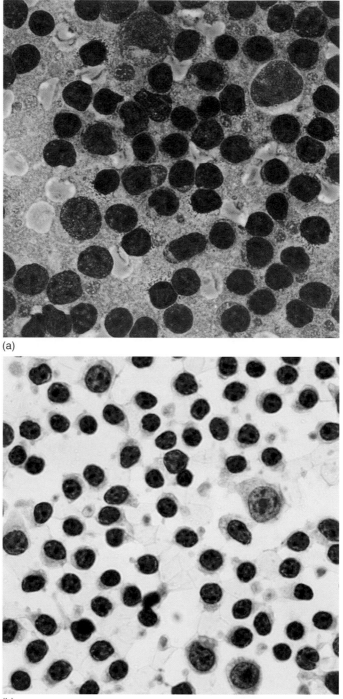

(a)

(b)

FIGURE 16.2. (*Continued*)

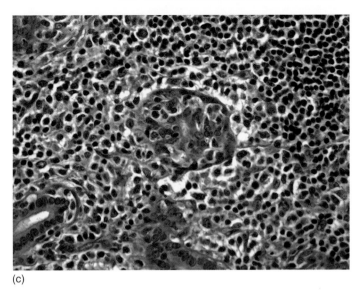

(c)

FIGURE 16.2. Marginal zone lymphoma of mucosa-associated lymphoid tissue. (a) A poly-morphous population of small- and medium-sized and occasional large lymphoid cells and plasma cells are observed. Frequent lymphoglandular bodies are noted (Diff-Quik, 1000×). (b) Frequent plasmacytoid lymphocytes and occasional plasma cells are observed (Papanicolaou, 1000×). (c) MALT lymphoma of parotid gland showing predominantly small- to medium-sized lymphoid cells and a formation of lymphoepithelial lesion (center; hematoxylin and eosin, 400×).

histologic sections; however, the transformation to diffuse large B-cell lymphoma should not be entertained unless one encounters sheets of large lymphoid cells.

The neoplastic cells of marginal zone lymphoma express CD20, CD19, and monoclonal immunoglobulin light chains. CD5, CD10, and cyclin D1 are absent. The coexpression of CD43 antigen on B cells is supportive of the diagnosis of MALT lymphoma. In cases with a significant colonization of follicles, the absence of the BCL2 protein on residual germinal center lympho-cytes can help in the differentiation between MALT and follicular lymphoma.

Numerous studies addressed the application of molecular studies as an aid in the diagnosis of MALT lymphoma. Because the clonal immunoglobulin heavy chain gene rearrangements also can be found in benign lymphoepithelial lesions in Sjogren syndrome patients, they cannot be used as a definitive confirmation of MALT lymphoma. Salivary gland MALT lymphomas fre-quently have been shown to harbor t(14;18)(q32;q21), and trisomies of chromosomes 3 and 18.

16.3.4   Cytologic Differential Diagnosis

The diagnosis and subclassification of low-grade lymphomas can be challen-ging when relying solely on cytologic examination. Table 16.3 provides

TABLE 16.3. Differential diagnosis of MALT lymphoma	
Major differential diagnosis	Clues to make the distinction
Lymphoepithelial sialoadenitis, autoimmune sialoadenitis	In addition to polymorphous lymphoid population, sialoadenitis shows aggregates of ductal epithelial cells. Oncocytes can be encountered. Definitive differentiation from MALT lymphoma is based on the demonstration of clonal lymphoid population by IHC or flow cytometry
Chronic sclerosing sialoadenitis (Kuttner tumor)	Kuttner tumor shows epithelial cells and stromal fragments with fibroblasts, features not frequently observed in MALT lymphoma. The demonstration of IgG4 positivity by IHC helps to solidify the diagnosis of Kuttner tumor
Lymphoepithelial cyst	Even though a mixed lymphoid population can be observed in lymphoepithelial cysts, the presence of foamy histiocytes, hemosiderin laden macrophages, tingible body macrophages, mucus, and proteinaceous material, which are not present in MALT lymphomas, are important diagnostic hints
Intraparotid lymph node	The presence of frequent tingible body macrophages and the paucity of plasma cells/plasmacytoid lymphocytes indicates the reactive lymphoid population
Warthin's tumor	A reactive lymphoid population including tingible body macrophages is accompanied by oncocytes and cystic fluid. Oncocytic change is observed rarely in MALT lymphoma
Malignant neoplasms with rich lymphocytic proliferation (e.g., acinic cell carcinoma, lymphoepithelial carcinoma)	The identification of acinic cells and large epithelial cells supports the diagnosis of nonlymphoid malignancy
Lymphomas with plasmacytic differentiation	Only rare cases of low-grade lymphomas with plasmacytic differentiation are encountered in salivary glands. The definitive subclassification requires correlation with clinical information and immunophenotypic features (IHC or flow cytometry)

several items for the differential diagnosis of MALT lymphoma. The cytology of lymphocyte-rich lesions has a low predictive value; thus, it has been suggested that a finding of a predominant lymphocyte population on FNA should prompt further evaluation with histologic examination. The addition of immunophenotyping aids significantly in the differential diagnosis between reactive conditions and neoplastic lymphoid proliferation and helps to limit differential diagnosis to select lymphoma subtypes. Nevertheless, the immunophenotyping does not circumvent the need for a histologic correlation in all cases.

The challenges in cytologic evaluation of lymphocyte-rich lesions stem from the fact that MALT lymphomas occurring in salivary glands exhibit the range of cell maturation/differentiation often observed in benign lymphoid proliferations. A heterogeneous population of small- and medium-sized lymphocytes, plasma cells, and immunoblasts typically is present in lymphoepithelial sialadenitis/benign lymphoepithelial lesion (LES), including autoimmune sialadenitis, chronic sclerosing sialadenitis (Kuttner tumor), HIV-related and nonimmunodeficiency-associated lymphoepithelial cysts, intraparotid lymph node, and to lesser degree, in chronic or granulomatous sialadenitis. In LES, in addition to an abundant heterogeneous lymphoid population, one might encounter fragments of epimyoepithelial islands, three-dimensional aggregates of ductal epithelial cells infiltrated by lymphocytes. Oncocytes also can be present. Depending on the stage of the disease, in chronic sclerosing sialadenitis, the fine needle aspirate smear can show variable components of ductal and epithelial cells, chronic inflammation, and stromal fragments with fibroblasts. If the lymphoplasmacytic component is significant and the cell block is available, then the staining for IgG4 immunostain helps to support the diagnosis of Kuttner tumor. The IgG4 immunohistochemical stain also should be considered in cases with a lymphoplasmacytic infiltrate in regional lymph nodes draining salivary gland tumors, as IgG4-positive interfollicular plasmacytosis has been described in Kuttner tumor. Similarly, the FNA smear of a lymphoepithelial cyst can show a mixed population of lymphocytes, foamy macrophages, tingible body macrophages, plasma cells, lymphohistiocytic aggregates, and occasionally hemosiderin-laden macrophages, mucus, proteinaceous material, and sparse epithelial cells. Squamous cells and ciliated epithelium can be present with only rare normal salivary gland cells. On the contrary, the aspiration of an intraparotid lymph node yields a rich lymphocytic population with scattered tingible body macrophages and occasionally with normal salivary gland epithelium. The epimyoepithelial islands are not observed when aspirating an intraparotid lymph node. The presence of tingible body macrophages favors a reactive process. The demonstration of a significant clonal lymphoid population, most commonly by flow cytometry, is supportive of the diagnosis of MALT lymphoma and occasionally also can provide additional information regarding lymphoma subclassification. The molecular studies for IgH gene rearrangements have demonstrated monoclonal populations in Sjogren syndrome-associated lymphoid proliferations and other autoimmune conditions and are not helpful in differential diagnosis between reactive lymphoid lesions and lymphoma.

Neoplastic lesions, both solid tumors with significant lymphoid component, such as Warthin's tumor, lymphadenoma, lymphoepithelial carcinoma, and lymphomas, are also considered in the differential diagnosis of MALT lymphoma. The aspiration of Warthin's tumor yields a variable amount of cystic fluid, characteristic oncocytes, and may include a rich lymphoid background. When a heterogeneous lymphoid population with tingible body macrophages is accompanied by oncocytes, the diagnosis of Warthin's tumor should be considered. Of note, acinic cell carcinoma occasionally can have a significant lymphoid infiltrate, and acinic cells can resemble oncocytes. Careful examination of Papanicolaou and Diff-Quik stains helps to differentiate acinic cells from oncocytes. Lymphadenoma is a rare benign neoplasm occurring in both pediatric and adult populations. In addition to cystic fluid, the aspiration can show epithelial cells and a rich reactive lymphoid background. Lymphoepithelial carcinoma is a rare malignancy of salivary glands. Large epithelial cells are present in a rich, mixed lymphoid background including small lymphocytes and plasma cells. Elements of reactive follicles also can be observed. Low-grade lymphomas other than MALT lymphoma are rare and, thus only rarely will be included in differential diagnosis. Small B-cell lymphomas with plasmacytic differentiation like lymphoplasmacytic lymphoma (LPL) most closely resemble MALT lymphoma. LPL consists of a heterogeneous population of small lymphocytes, plasmacytoid lymphocytes, and plasma cells. The clinical presentation, hyperviscosity with an IgM monoclonal protein (M component), and the evidence of primary involvement of bone marrow are important diagnostic indicators. Other low-grade lymphomas, like chronic lymphocytic leukemia/small lymphocytic lymphoma (CLL/SLL), follicular lymphoma (FL), and mantle cell lymphoma (MCL) show more monomorphic lymphoid populations devoid of plasma cells. CLL/SLL consist of a monotonous population of small lymphoid cells with scant cytoplasm. Low-grade FL has a predominant population of monotonous small-cleaved centrocytes with occasional large centroblasts. Similarly, MCL shows monotonous medium-sized lymphoid cells with irregular nuclear outlines and paucity of large transformed lymphocytes. Definitive subclassification of low-grade lymphomas requires immunophenotyping, either by immunohistochemistry of a cell block or by flow cytometry. The expression of CD5 and CD23 together with characteristic low-intensity CD20 and immunoglobulin light chain is typical for CLL/SLL. CD10 and BCL6 are positive in FL, and cyclin D1 expression is diagnostic of MCL. Not infrequently, if these typical immunophenotypic features are not evident on cytologic material, then excision is required for definitive subclassification.

16.3.5 Treatment and Prognosis

MALT lymphoma is an indolent disease with a chronic clinical course. It usually remains localized to the salivary glands. Surgical excision or local radiation therapy provide prolonged remission or cure in most cases. Transformation to diffuse large B-cell lymphoma is rare.

16.4 FOLLICULAR LYMPHOMA

16.4.1 Introduction

Follicular lymphoma (FL), along with diffuse large B-cell lymphoma, is one of the most common malignant lymphomas in the Western hemisphere. It originates from germinal center cells and in most cases has a follicular architecture. Depending on the proportion of centrocytes and centroblasts, follicular lymphomas are classified as low and high grade. This distinction is clinically relevant because the low-grade cases represent an indolent incurable disease, and the high-grade follicular lymphomas require more aggressive treatment.

16.4.2 Clinical Features

FL occurs predominantly in the adult population with a slight female predominance. Low-grade FL (histologic grade 1–2) presents in most cases as a disseminated disease involving peripheral and central lymph nodes, spleen, and bone marrow. A variety of extranodal sites can be involved both as an extension of disseminated disease and as a primary presentation. Skin, gastrointestinal tract, and ocular adnexa have been cited most frequently as primary extranodal sites. Primary FL of salivary glands, including submandibular and parotid glands, is less frequent than MALT lymphoma. These cases either can be limited to the involvement of a salivary gland and regional cervical lymph nodes or can be disseminated at the time of diagnosis.

16.4.3 Cytologic Features with Histologic Correlates

In most cases, cytologic features are a reflection of histologic presentation. The fine needle aspirations are highly cellular with numerous lymphocytes. The predominance of small-to-medium-sized lymphocytes with cleaved nuclei is observed in low-grade FL (histological grade 1–2; Figures 16.2a and b, Table 16.1). High-grade (histologic grade 3) FL shows frequent large lymphoid cells (larger than a nucleus of a histiocyte) with round to oval nuclei, smooth nuclear membrane, and at least two medium-sized nucleoli located peripherally in the nucleus. In most cases, grade-3 FL resembles diffuse large B-cell lymphoma. Regardless of the grade, lymphoglandular bodies are frequent. The definitive subclassification and differentiation of FL from other types of low-grade lymphomas requires demonstration of follicular center cell immunophenotype as described in the following paragraphs.

The evaluation of FNA smears does not allow the determination of the growth pattern (follicular vs. diffuse), which is an important component of the diagnosis, particularly in grade-3 FL. It has been shown that patients with grade-3 FL and more than 25% of the diffuse pattern (areas of diffuse large B-cell lymphoma) have a more adverse prognosis when compared with patients with a purely follicular pattern.

Histologically, numerous closely spaced follicles replace the normal nodal architecture (Figure 16.3c). The mantle zone and the intrafollicular polarization, usually observed in reactive secondary follicles, are not preserved in FL. Medium-sized lymphoid cells with angular or cleaved nuclei (centrocytes) and a variable number of large lymphoid cells (centroblasts) are scattered randomly in neoplastic follicles. Based on the frequency of centroblasts in the follicles, FL is classified as grade 1–2 (low grade, 0–15 centroblasts per high-power field) and grade 3 (more than 15 centroblasts per high-power field). Diffuse areas demonstrating more than 15 centroblasts per high-power field are designated as diffuse large B-cell lymphoma. Cases classified as grade-3 FL have a more aggressive clinical course. The finding of focal diffuse high-grade areas (i.e., diffuse large B-cell lymphoma) within otherwise predominantly follicular grade-3 FL is also of prognostic significance.

The immunophenotype reflects the follicle center cell origin. Pan-B cell markers (CD19, CD20) are present along with the coexpression of CD10,

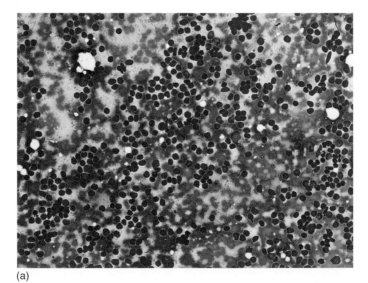

(a)

FIGURE 16.3. (*Continued*)

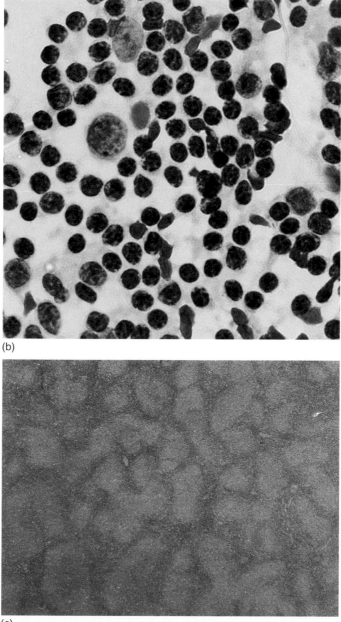

(b)

(c)

FIGURE 16.3. Follicular lymphoma. (**a**) The lymphoid population in low-grade FL is more monotonous than in MALT lymphomas. Small- to medium-sized centrocytes with cleaved/irregular nuclei are accompanied by only rare large centroblasts (Diff-Quik, 400×). (**b**) The number of centroblasts (on the left of center), large lymphoid cells with scant cytoplasm and peripherally placed nucleoli, is dependent on the grade of FL (Papanicolaou, 1000×). (**c**) Histologic sections show numerous back-to-back follicles (hematoxylin and eosin, 40×)

BCL-6, and clonal surface immunoglobulin. In contrast to reactive follicles, neoplastic cells express BCL2 protein because of the t(14;18)(q32;q21), which places the BCL2 gene under a promoter of the immunoglobulin heavy chain gene. This cytogenetic abnormality is present in 95% of cases and can be demonstrated by fluorescent in situ hybridization on cytospin/FNA smear.

16.4.4   Cytologic Differential Diagnosis

The cytologic differential diagnosis for follicular lymphoma includes both reactive conditions and benign and malignant neoplasms (Table 16.4). Immunophenotyping, performed either by flow cytometry of FNA or by immunohistochemistry on the cell block, are essential to exclude reactive lymphoid proliferations and aid in lymphoma subclassification. Similar to MALT lymphoma, any lesion accompanied by a marked lymphocytic

TABLE 16.4. Differential diagnosis of follicular lymphoma	
Major differential diagnosis	Clues to make the distinction
Reactive lymphoid proliferations associated with autoimmune conditions, lymphoepithelial cysts, intraparotid lymph nodes, Warthin's tumor, and select salivary gland malignancies	See differential diagnosis of MALT lymphoma
MALT lymphoma	Most common differential diagnosis. The lymphoid population in MALT lymphoma is more polymorphous, whereas low-grade FL shows a monomorphic population of centrocytes with only rare large cells centroblasts. A significant population of plasma cells and plasmacytoid lymphocytes is absent in classical cases of low-grade FL
Diffuse large B-cell lymphoma	DLBCL is cytologically and immunohistochemically indistinguishable from high-grade FL. Both show a predominance of large lymphoid cells and can be of germinal center cell immunophenotype. Open biopsy is required to demonstrate the growth pattern—follicular versus diffuse

infiltrate can resemble low-grade FL. Typically, cases of lymphoepithelial sialadenitis and chronic sclerosing sialadenitis show polymorphous lymphocytic proliferation comprising small, medium-sized, and large transformed lymphocytes, plasma cells, and tingible body macrophages with a background of benign epithelial cells. The cytologic features of lymphoepithelial cysts, intraparotid lymph nodes, Warthin's tumor, lymphadenoma, and lymphoepithelial carcinoma are discussed in detail in the MALT lymphoma section. The most important cytologic features in support of the diagnosis of low-grade FL are cellular FNA with a homogenous population of small-to-medium-sized lymphocytes with cleaved nuclei, rare large lymphoid cells, and a lack of tingible body macrophages. Immunophenotypic studies demonstrating the monoclonal B-cell population and presence of markers associated with a follicular center cell origin are required for subclassification in most cases.

The main differential diagnosis for grade-3 FL is diffuse large B-cell lymphoma. In a proportion of cases, the cytologic features of immunoblastic or plasmablastic differentiation can aid in the subclassification. However, most frequently, the distinction between the two can be challenging or not possible even with the support of immunophenotyping because of an overlap in surface marker expression. In these cases, final classification of the lesion will require an open biopsy.

16.4.5 Treatment and Prognosis

Low-grade follicular lymphoma developing in salivary glands is an indolent disease with a prolonged clinical course. Both local radiation therapy and a combination of radiation and multiagent chemotherapy are used. The prognosis is dependent on the stage of the disease (localized vs. disseminated) and the grade (grade 1–2 vs. grade 3).

16.5 DIFFUSE LARGE B-CELL LYMPHOMA

16.5.1 Introduction

The defining feature of DLBCL is the large size of neoplastic cells and diffuse growth pattern. DLBCL is one of the most common lymphoid neoplasms and can present as a primary disease or develop as a transformation of preexisting low-grade lymphoma. It can originate at any differentiation stage of mature B-cell.

The 2008 WHO classification defines several subtypes of DLBCL based on the morphologic features, clinical presentation, and an association with infectious agents. Consequently, DLBCL can differ significantly in cytologic appearance and immunophenotype.

16.5.2 Clinical Features

Overall, DLBCL is more common in elderly patients with median age in the seventh decade; however, the age distribution is dependent on the subtype. DLBCL not otherwise classified occurs most frequently in elderly patients, whereas other subtypes can affect younger age groups. The sites of involvement and the extent of the disease at diagnosis are related to the histologic type. Salivary gland DLBCL primarily develops from the preexisting MALT lymphoma; however, in rare instances, it may represent a primary diagnosis.

16.5.3 Cytologic Features with Histologic Correlates

Most commonly, the FNA of DLBCL is cellular with a monomorphic population of large lymphoid cells and prominent lymphoglandular bodies (Figure 16.4a, Table 16.1). The lymphoid population is usually noncohesive; however, in individual cases, lymphocytes can aggregate (Figure 16.4b). The size of cells is larger than that of a nucleus of a histiocyte. The nuclear-to-cytoplasmic ratios are variable. Cytoplasm is usually basophilic and can contain vacuoles. The nuclear outlines can be irregular and chromatic variably condensed. Occasionally, nuclei are multilobated. Nucleoli can be prominent. Apoptotic debris with associated tingible body macrophages and necrosis can be present. The admixture of small lymphocytes and other cells

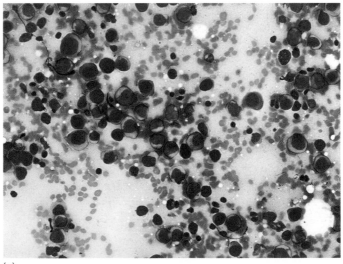

(a)

FIGURE 16.4. (*Continued*)

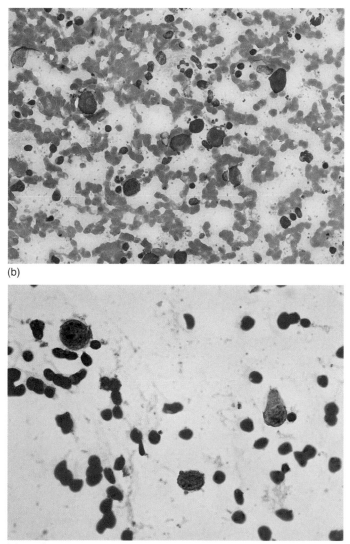

(b)

(c)

FIGURE 16.4. (*Continued*)

such as granulocytes is variable and dependent on the subtype of DLBCL (Figure 16.4c)

Histologic sections show a diffuse proliferation of large lymphoid cells infiltrating through gland parenchyma. In DLBCL resulting from preexisting MALT lymphoma, a variable admixture of small and medium lymphocytes and plasma cells is observed. Primary DLBCL of a salivary gland usually consists of a monomorphic population of large lymphoid cells. Even though

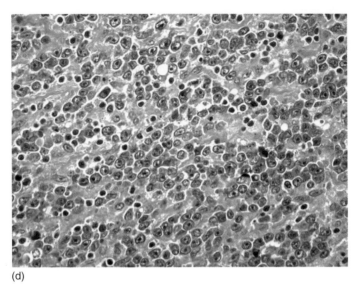

(d)

FIGURE 16.4. Diffuse large B-cell lymphoma. (**a**) Cellular FNA smear with frequent discohesive large lymphoid cells. Small lymphocytes can be present in the background (Diff-Quik,
500×). (**b**) DLBCL with large lymphoid cells and frequent background small lymphocytes and
granulocytes (Diff-Quik, 500×). (**c**) FNA smear with rare large lymphoid cells of DLBCL
(Papanicolaou stain, 1000×). (**d**) Histologic sections of DLBCL show sheets of large lymphoid
cells (hematoxylin and eosin, 400×).

the histologic features in most cases are diagnostic of large-cell lymphoma,
immunohistochemical studies are essential to confirm the B-cell origin and in
select cases to differentiate DLBCL from nonlymphoid neoplasms. As in other
B-cell lymphomas, pan-B-cell antigens are expressed. DLBCL can derive from
a variety of stages in B-cell development, hence the coexpression of other
markers such as CD5, CD10, BCL-6, CD30, and CD138.

16.5.4   Differential Diagnosis

The differential diagnosis includes other lymphomas comprising predominantly large lymphoid cells such as select T-cell lymphomas, anaplastic large
cell lymphoma, and rarely cHL (Table 16.5). Poorly differentiated carcinomas,
small-cell carcinomas, and malignant melanomas also are included in the
differential diagnosis depending on their relative frequencies in the salivary
glands.

16.5.5   Treatment and Prognosis

DLBCL is an aggressive neoplasm. Usually, patients are treated with radiation and multiagent combination therapy such as R-CHOP. The recurrence
rate is high.

TABLE 16.5. Differential diagnosis of diffuse large B-cell lymphoma	
Major differential diagnosis	Clues to make the distinction
Other lymphomas consisting predominantly of large cells (e.g., high-grade FL or anaplastic large cell lymphoma)	Distinction requires detailed immunophenotype either by flow cytometry of FNA or by IHC of cell block, and frequently open biopsy
Nonlymphoid neoplasms (e.g., poorly differentiated carcinoma, small cell carcinoma, or malignant melanoma)	DLBCL infrequently can show cell clustering resembling a solid tumor; cytologic features can show a significant overlap, and nuclear streaking can be present in DLBCL. On the contrary, a select solid tumor may show a discohesive pattern on FNA smears. Lymphoglandular bodies characteristically are observed in lymphoma cases and are absent in solid tumors. Clinical information and IHC including the CD45 (LCA) antigen are helpful in the diagnosis

16.6 PLASMA CELL NEOPLASMS

16.6.1 Introduction

Plasma cell neoplasms are extremely rare in salivary glands. They consist of a monoclonal proliferation of plasma cells and can present as a localized salivary gland mass (plasmacytoma) or as a disseminated process including bone marrow involvement (plasma cell myeloma).

16.6.2 Clinical Features

Soft-tissue plasmacytoma usually presents in the head and neck in the upper respiratory tract. Salivary gland involvement has been reported rarely. Patients usually present with symptoms related to a local mass effect. Plasma cell myeloma with extramedullary plasmacytoma of a salivary gland can occur; thus, in all cases of plasmacytoma, a careful staging including a bone marrow exam should be performed.

16.6.3 Cytologic Features with Histologic Correlates

FNA usually generates a cellular specimen rich in cytologically atypical plasma cells, which can form loose sheets. Plasma cells have an abundant basophilic cytoplasm, perinuclear hof (Golgi area), and eccentric nucleus with clock-faced chromatin (Figure 16.5a and b, Table 16.1). Immature plasma cells have prominent nucleoli and less clumped chromatin. Atypical plasma cells are enlarged with an increased nuclear-to-cytoplasmic ratio

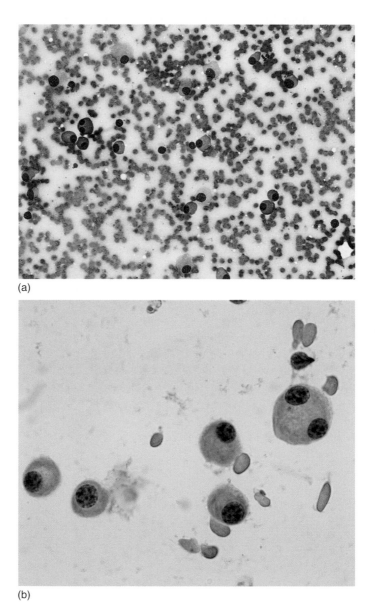

(a)

(b)

FIGURE 16.5. (*Continued*)

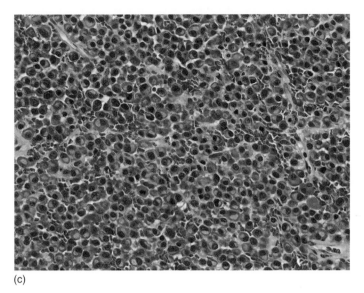

(c)

FIGURE 16.5. Plasmacytoma. (a) Frequent plasma cells with mild cytologic atypia (binu-cleated forms and cells with increased nuclear cytoplasmic ratio; Diff-Quik 500×). (b) Similar cytologic features shown on Papanicolaou stain (Papanicolaou, 1000×). (c) Sheets of cytolo-gically atypical plasma cells (hematoxylin and eosin, 500×).

and/or multinucleation. Bizzare and immature forms are frequently observed in cases of disseminated plasma cell myeloma.

Histologically, sheets of plasma cells, frequently with cytologic atypia, are noted (Figure 16.5c). Neoplastic plasma cells show an immunophenotype similar to that of their normal counterparts. At this terminal stage of differentiation, pan-B-cell markers, CD19 and CD20, and surface immunoglo-bulin chains are absent in most cases. Plasma cells are positive for CD138, high-density CD38 antigen, and cytoplasmic immunoglobulins. The clonality of plasma cell proliferation is demonstrated best using immunohistochemical stains or flow cytometry for immunoglobulin light chains (Kappa or Lambda).

16.6.4 Differential Diagnosis

Plasma cell neoplasms consist of sheets of plasma cells. Therefore, benign and malignant lesions with plasmacytic differentiation are important differ-ential diagnoses (Table 16.6). Autoimmune sialadenitis and chronic scleros-ing sialadenitis can present with a rich lymphoplasmacytic proliferation with numerous plasma cells. Close attention to the presence of a background lymphoid population along with the demonstration of polyclonal plasma cells by either flow cytometry or immunohistochemistry is essential for

TABLE 16.6. Differential diagnosis of plasma cell neoplasms

Major differential diagnosis	Clues to make the distinction
Reactive conditions with significant plasma cell component (e.g., autoimmune sialoadenitis)	The differential diagnosis of these two lesions is rarely an issue because of an admixture of lymphocytes in reactive conditions
Lymphomas with plasma cell differentiation (e.g., MALT lymphoma or plasmablastic/immunoblastic lymphomas)	MALT lymphoma demonstrates a spectrum of lymphoid cells including small- and medium-sized lymphocytes, plasmacytoid lymphocytes, and plasma cells. This spectrum is not observed in plasma cell neoplasms. In rare cases of MALT lymphoma with extreme plasma cell differentiation, open biopsy may be required to show residual follicles present in MALT lymphoma and absent in plasma cell neoplasms. Cells of high-grade lymphomas of plasmablastic or immunoblastic subtype can resemble atypical and immature plasma cells of plasma cell myeloma. The correlation with clinical information (widespread lytic lesions) and demonstration of bone marrow involvement are required to differentiate these entities
Nonhematopoietic malignancies (e.g., malignant melanoma and some carcinomas)	May resemble atypical or immature plasma cells because of nuclear cytoplasmic polarity and a discohesive pattern on FNA smear. Clinical correlation and IHC (S-100, HMB45, CD138/kappa/lambda, and Cytokeratins) help in the differential diagnosis

definitive diagnosis. In such cases, adequate sampling with sufficient FNA/cell block material is critical.

A proportion of low-grade B-cell lymphomas show a significant plasma cell differentiation. Most commonly, marginal zone/MALT lymphomas have a plasmacytic component, which in extreme cases is a predominant finding on cytologic examination. In these rare cases, open biopsy demonstrating residual or colonized reactive follicles is helpful in diagnosing MALT lymphoma. Rarely, small lymphocytic lymphoma and follicular lymphoma can show an abundance of plasma cells. Similarly, an immunophenotype of background lymphoid population aids in the diagnosis of these rare salivary gland lymphomas.

16.6.5 Treatment and Prognosis

Treatment of plasmacytoma usually includes local surgical excision and adjuvant radiotherapy. A risk is present of local recurrence; however, the progression to disseminated plasma cell myeloma is rare. The role of adjuvant chemotherapy is unclear.

RECOMMENDED READINGS

Chang KT, Chadha NK, Leung R, Shago M, Phillips MJ, Thorner PS. Lymphadenoma-case report of a rare salivary gland tumor in childhood. Pediatr Dev Pathol 2009. Forthcoming.

Chhieng DC, Cangiarella JF, Cohen JM. Fine-needle aspiration cytology of lymphoproliferative lesions involving the major salivary glands. Am J Clin Pathol 2000;113:563–571.

Cohen EG, Patel SG, Lin O, Boyle JO, Kraus DH, Singh B, Wong RJ, Shah JP, Shaha AR. Fine-needle aspiration biopsy of salivary gland lesions in a selected patient population. Arch Otolaryngol Head Neck Surg 2004;130:773–778.

Crapanzano JP, Lin O. Cytologic findings of marginal zone lymphoma. Cancer 2003;25:301–309.

Ellis GL. Lymphoid lesions of salivary glands: malignant and benign. Med Oral Patol Oral Cir Bucal 2007;12:E479–85.

Gonzalez-Garcia J, Ghufoor K, Sandhu G, Thorpe PA, Hadley J. Primary extramedullary plasmacytoma of the parotid gland: a case report and review of the literature. J Laryngol Otol 1998;112:179 181.

Ihrler S, Harrison JD. Mikulicz's disease and Mikulicz's syndrome: analysis of the original case report of 1892 in the light of current knowledge identifies a MALT lymphoma. Oral Surg Oral Med Oral Pathol Oral Radiol Endod 2005;100: 334–339.

Kojima M, Miyawaki S, Takada S, Kashiwabara K, Igarashi T, Nakamura S. Lymphoplasmacytic infiltrate of regional lymph nodes in Kuttner's tumor (chronic sclerosing sialadenitis): a report of 3 cases. Int J Surg Pathol 2008;16:263–268.

Kojima M, Shimizu K, Nishikawa M, Tamaki Y, Ito H, Tsukamoto N, Masawa N. Primary salivary gland lymphoma among Japanese: A clinicopathological study of 30 cases. Leuk Lymphoma 2007;48:1793–1798.

Landgren O, MacDonald AP, Tani E, Tani E, Czader M, Grimfors G, Skoog L, Ost A, Wedelin C, Axdorph U, Svedmyr E, Björkholm M. A prospective comparison of fine-needle aspiration cytology and histopathology in the diagnosis and classification of lymphomas. 2004;5:69–76.

Masuda M, Segawa Y, Joe AK, Hirakawa N, Komune S. A case of primary Hodgkin's lymphoma of the parotid gland. Auris Nasus Larynx 2008;34:440–442.

Nakamura S, Ichimura K, Sato Y, Nakamura S, Nakamine H, Inagaki H, Sadahira Y, Ohshima K, Sakugawa S, Kondo E, Yanai H, Ohara N, Yoshino T. Follicular lymphoma frequently originates in the salivary gland. Pathol Int 2006;56:576–583.

Swerdlow, SH, Campo E, Harris NL, Jaffe ES, Pileri SA, Stein H, Thiele J, Vardiman JW. WHO Classification of Tumours of Haematopoietic and Lymphoid Tissues. 4th ed. Lyon, France: WHO Press; 2008.

Yencha MW. Primary parotid gland Hodgkin's lymphoma. Ann Otol Rhinol Laryngol 2002;111:338–342.

Zhang C, Cohen JM, Cangiarella JF, Waisman J, McKenna BJ, Chhieng DC. Fine-needle aspiration of secondary neoplasms involving the salivary glands. A report of 36 cases. Am J Clin Pathol 2000;113:21–28.

CHAPTER 17

METASTASES AND RARE PRIMARY NEOPLASMS OF SALIVARY GLANDS

MOUSA A. AL-ABBADI, MD, FIAC

17.1 INTRODUCTION

As mentioned in Chapter 1, the recent World Health Organization (WHO) classification includes a large list of tumors that are basically very rare. Cytological recognition and appropriate classification based solely on the grounds of aspiration smears is difficult. An easier task is determining a categorical diagnosis or differential diagnosis. In many of these cases, the final diagnosis will be made on histological evaluation after surgical excision. Metastasis to salivary glands is also rare but can occur and pose diagnostic challenges. The first part of this chapter will cover metastatic tumors, and the second portion will include a brief description of each of these rare primary tumors. Most reports in cytologic and fine needle aspiration literature about these entities are in the form of case reports.

17.2 METASTATIC TUMORS TO SALIVARY GLANDS

Salivary glands are an unusual site for metastases. However, the glands and its associated lymph nodes sometimes can be involved with metastatic tumors and consequently pose diagnostic challenges specifically to answer the question of primary versus metastasis. Metastases to salivary glands comprise approximately 5% of all malignant tumors of salivary glands, and they are more frequent in the parotid gland. If a history of malignancy is

Salivary Gland Cytology: A Color Atlas, Edited by Mousa A. Al-Abbadi
Copyright © 2011 Wiley-Blackwell

known, then the task is usually easier, and the best approach is to compare the morphological appearance of both neoplasms. However, if the patient presents with salivary gland malignancy that could be secondary with no prior known history, then the pathologist task is harder and finding the primary site needs thorough clinical and radiological work up. In these circumstances, taking a short screening history and a head and neck examination during the fine needle aspiration (FNA) procedure may unveil a potential source. Carcinoma and melanoma in and around the head and neck region may be found. The most common sources of metastasis to salivary glands are head and neck carcinoma, mostly squamous cell carcinoma (Figure 17.1a–c) followed by melanoma (Figure 17.2a–e). The parotid gland is the most common gland involved, and most commonly, the primary site is in the head and neck region. However, the source of metastasis to the submandibular glands is more frequently from distant sites. Any organ can send metastasis to a salivary gland, but lung (predominantly small cell carcinoma), kidney, and breast are among the most common. In rare occasions, the primary site may not be identified. Metastases are thought to occur primarily through lymphatic spread and to a lesser extent occur by direct extension or hematogenous spread. It is believed that up to 75% of parotid metastases may represent a secondary tumor to an intraparotid lymph node from nearby malignancy.

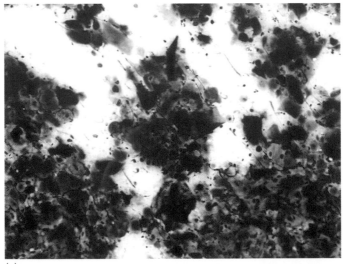

(a)

FIGURE 17.1. (*Continued*)

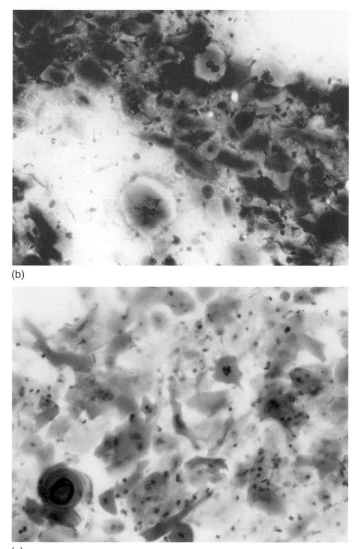

(b)

(c)

FIGURE 17.1. (**a**) Aspirate smears from a parotid mass in a patient who had a previously confirmed diagnosis of keratinizing squamous cell carcinoma of the base of the tongue. Clusters of epithelial cells are observed at low power (Diff Quik, 200×). (**b**) A higher view demonstrating the atypical large cells with a hard cytoplasm characteristic of squamous cell carcinoma (Diff Quik, 400×). (**c**) Clusters of keratinizing squamous cell carcinoma are obvious on a Papanicolaou stain. No further diagnostic work up was needed (Papanicolaou, 400×).

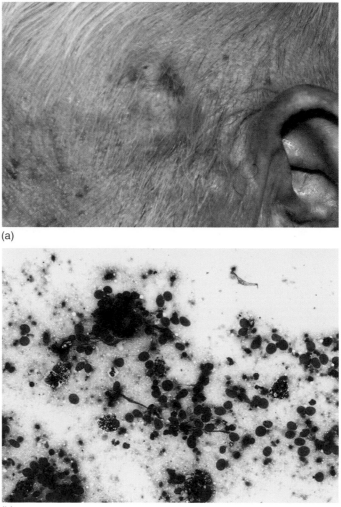

(a)

(b)

FIGURE 17.2. (*Continued*)

17.3 RARE PRIMARY NEOPLASMS OF SALIVARY GLANDS

17.3.1 Canalicular Adenoma

Despite the fact that this neoplasm can be categorized as a pleomorphic or a monomorphic adenoma variant (epithelial-rich pleomorphic adenoma), many investigators believe that it deserves to be dealt with as a separate entity because it has unique clinicopathological features. This tumor involves the upper lip in most cases with few cases affecting the buccal

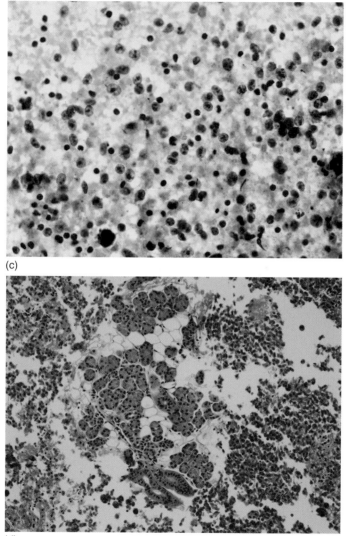

(c)

(d)

FIGURE 17.2. (*Continued*)

mucosa. It rarely involves major salivary glands. Clinically, the peak incidence is in the seventh decade, and it affects females more than males. Although most cases are solitary, some cases can be multiple. Making the specific diagnosis of "canalicular adenoma" by fine needle aspiration is not easy. However, the smears are usually cellular and show benign-appearing cuboidal and columnar epithelium in cords. Cords comprising biepithelial cell layers (canaliculi) are characteristic (Figures 17.3a and b). In addition,

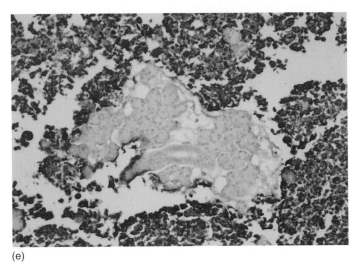

(e)

FIGURE 17.2. (**a**) A photomicrograph of a pigmented lesion on the left temple, the primary source of metastatic melanoma to the left parotid gland. The lesion was found immediately at the time of fine needle aspiration after evaluating the first pass that showed potential metastatic melanoma. (**b**) Smears from the parotid showing multiple medium size cells with an ovoid nucleus, some of which contain pigmented cytoplasm. While evaluating this smear and assuming a potential melanoma diagnosis, both the pathologist and the otolaryngologist examined the surrounding skin where a pigmented lesion was found just above the temple area (Diff Quik, 400×). (**c**) Smears from the previous case showing a predominance of single cells, some of which have pigmented cytoplasm, and ovoid-to-round nuclei with prominent nucleoli (Papanicolaou, 600×). (**d**) The cell block showed unremarkable salivary gland tissue surrounded by the malignant cells. Immunohistochemical stains on the cell block confirmed the diagnosis of melanoma (hematoxylin and eosin, 400×). (**e**) The tumor cells are immunoreactive for HMB-45 surrounding the negative unremarkable salivary gland tissue (HMB-45 immunostain on cell block, 200×).

thin stroma can be intermixed that sometimes can show globules reminiscent of adenoid cystic carcinoma globules (Figures 17.3c and d). However, these stromal globules are thin and not as darkly metachromatic as their adenoid cystic carcinoma counterparts. In addition, no cellular or nuclear atypia are present. The histological features are characteristic; the tumor is well circumscribed and sometimes encapsulated. Sections show cords of benign columnar and cuboidal epithelial cells in double layers with thin and slightly vascular stroma (Figure 17.3e). The stroma is not fibrillary and no myoepithelial cells are present; both are features that separate canalicular adenoma from classic pleomorphic adenoma.

17.3.2 Cystadenoma and Cystadenocarcinoma

These rare tumors are characterized by a predominant cystic growth by imaging (Figure 17.4a), gross examination, and a predominant bland

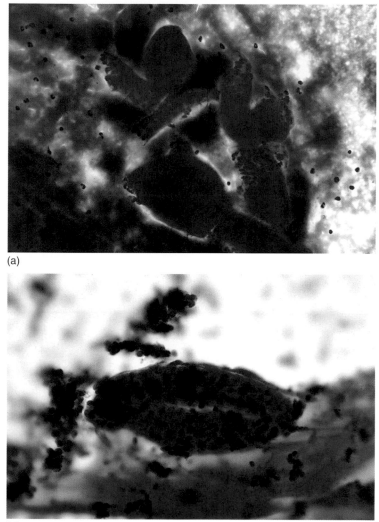

(a)

(b)

FIGURE 17.3. (*Continued*)

papillary morphology on cytological smears. Cystadenocarcinoma (also known as nonepidermoid mucous-producing adenopapillary carcinoma, malignant papillary cystadenoma, and low-grade papillary adenocarcinoma of the palate) is the malignant counterpart of cystadenoma. The cyst lining is epithelial and adenomatous ranging from intestinal-type epithelium to clear and occasional bland cuboidal. The only way to differentiate carcinoma from adenoma is with histological evidence of invasion either into the surrounding normal salivary gland epithelium or into the surrounding

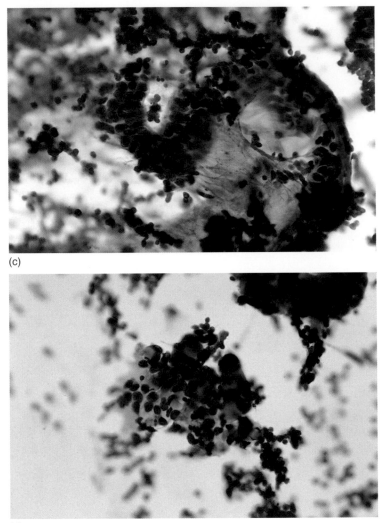

(c)

(d)

FIGURE 17.3. (*Continued*)

structures. Therefore, FNA smears of both will show similar features. Aspirate smears are moderately cellular and consist of papillary glandular clusters (Figure 17.4b) without the squamous or intermediate cells that characterize mucoepidermoid carcinoma. Occasional mucinous cells can be found, and in general, the nuclear morphology is bland (Figure 17.4c). The histological sections are multicystic and contain papillary structures lined by cuboidal or columnar cells (Figures 17.4d and e). Cystadenoma is benign

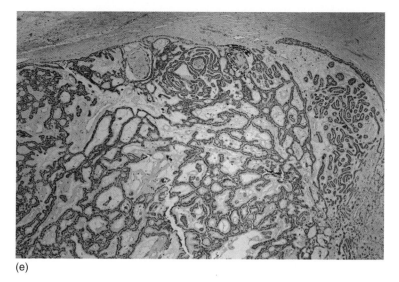

(e)

FIGURE 17.3. (**a**) A low-power view showing the double epithelial cords of bland columnar cells (Diff Quik, 200×). (**b**) A low-power view showing the double epithelial cords of bland columnar cells and a thin stroma shown at the bottom of the image (Papanicolaou, 200×). (**c**) A higher power view showing the double epithelial cords of bland columnar cells and a thin stroma, which can stream but is not fibrillary (Papanicolaou, 400×). (**d**) Sometimes the stroma seem globular and intermixed with the epithelial cells, raising the possibility of adenoid cystic carcinoma. However, the stroma is thin and not as dark (Papanicolaou, 400×). (**e**) The histological sections demonstrate well-circumscribed and encapsulated neoplasm with anastomosing cords comprising double epithelial cell layers and thin intervening stroma (hematoxylin and eosin, 40×). Courtesy of H. Cramer, Indiana University, Indianapolis, IN.

and is cured by complete surgical excision, whereas cystadenocarcinoma is a slow-growing, low-grade adenocarcinoma treated by a wide local excision of the involved gland. Metastasis and mortality from this carcinoma is unusual. Another entity that sometimes overlaps with these neoplasms is low-grade cribriform cystadenocarcinoma (also known as low-grade salivary duct carcinoma). This rare tumor resembles atypical ductal hyperplasia of the breast, and FNA smears may resemble those of cystadenocarcinoma and cystadenoma.

17.3.3   Sebaceous Adenoma and Sebaceous Carcinoma

Sebaceous adenoma is a benign, usually well-circumscribed neoplasm of bland sebaceous cells that lack cellular or nuclear atypia or pleomorphism. Histological examination shows clusters of sebaceous glands of variable size that frequently contain foci of squamous differentiation without infiltration of the surrounding tissue structures. The cells are bland with clear cytoplasm. In this tumor, fine needle aspirate smears may show cells

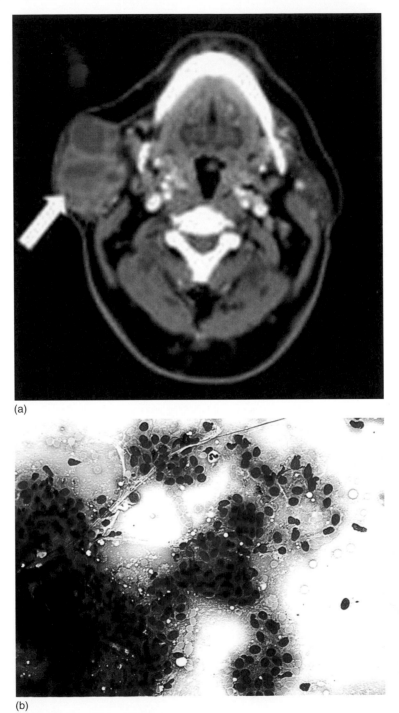

(a)

(b)

FIGURE 17.4. (*Continued*)

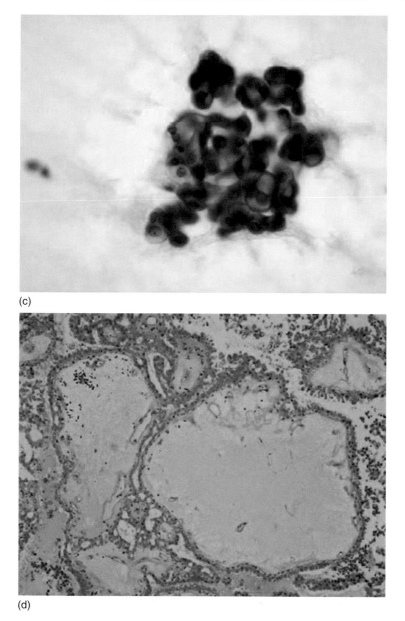

(c)

(d)

FIGURE 17.4. (*Continued*)

with clear cytoplasm and squamous cells, a combination that may lead to misinterpretation as mucoepidermoid carcinoma. On the contrary, sebaceous carcinoma will exhibit obvious features of malignancy both at the cellular and the architectural levels in which invasion and infiltration of

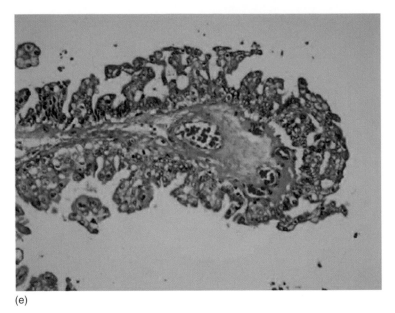

(e)

FIGURE 17.4. (**a**) Computerized tomography of the neck area, transverse section, showing a right parotid multicystic and well-circumscribed lesion (arrow). (**b**) Smears showing papillary clusters of polygonal and slightly elongate cells with clear cytoplasm and oval bland nuclei (May–Grünwald–Giemsa [MGG] stain, 400×). Courtesy of J. Klijanienko, Institut Curie, Paris, France. (**c**) A higher view of these cells in the papillae showing bland cells with abundant and focally vacuolated cytoplasm and round nuclei (Papanicolaou, 600×). Courtesy of N. Aloudah, King Khalid University Hospital, Riyadh, Saudi Arabia. (**d**) Histological section of the tumor showing multiple microcyts and papillae floating in a mucoid background (hematoxylin and eosin, 40×). Courtesy of N. Aloudah, King Khalid University Hospital, Riyadh, Saudi Arabia. (**e**) A higher view of the histological sections demonstrating the bland papillary structures lined by cuboidal cells with slightly vacuolated cytoplasm. This tumor showed stromal invasion in other areas justifying the diagnosis of low-grade papillary cystadenocarcinoma. Without invasion, papillary cystadenoma would be the correct diagnosis. The distinction is almost impossible on cytological aspirate smears (hematoxylin and eosin, 100×). Courtesy of N. Aloudah, King Khalid University Hospital, Riyadh, Saudi Arabia.

the surrounding tissue is evident. The cells can have squamous and sometimes basaloid differentiation making the diagnosis and classification of this tumor very difficult on fine needle aspiration smears.

17.3.4 Lymphadenoma (Sebaceous and Nonsebaceous)

These tumors are rare and affect mainly the parotid gland and are encapsulated or well circumscribed (Figure 17.5a) and consist of a collection of benign-appearing ducts and epithelium with a background of intense lymphoid cells and lymphoid follicles. If the epithelial cells contain obvious sebaceous glands, then it is called sebaceous lymphadenoma, and if it

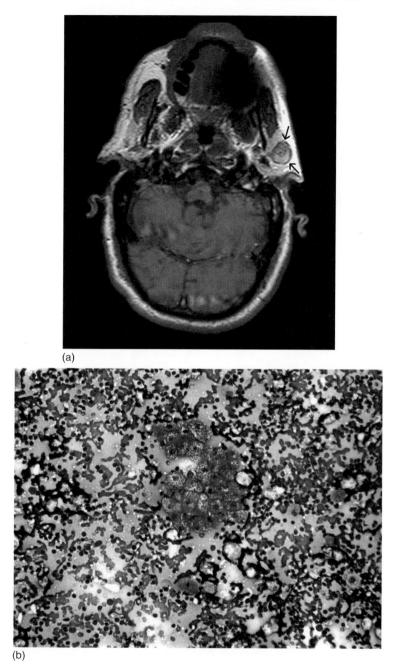

(a)

(b)

FIGURE 17.5. (*Continued*)

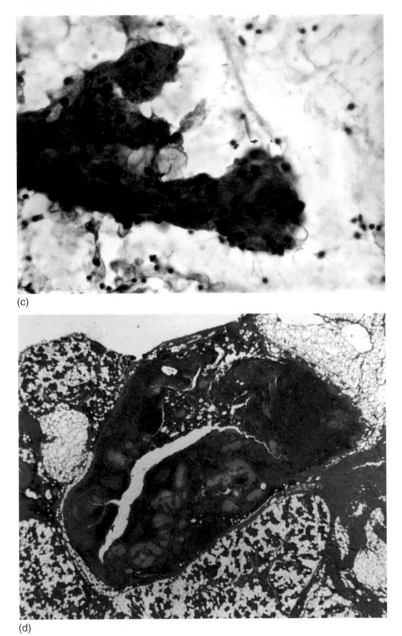

(c)

(d)

FIGURE 17.5. (*Continued*)

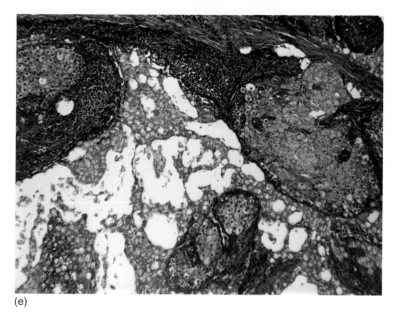

(e)

FIGURE 17.5. (**a**) Magnetic resonance image showing a well-circumscribed lesion (arrow) in the superficial lobe of the left parotid gland. Courtesy of I. Zak, Wayne State University, Detroit, MI. (**b**) The smears show benign and bland sebaceous cells in clusters that are surrounded by numerous small mature-seeming lymphocytes (Diff Quik, 200×). Courtesy of J. Feng and S. Bandyopadhyay, Wayne State University, Detroit, MI. (**c**) At a high power, this smear shows benign and bland clusters of sebaceous cells surrounded by small mature lymphocytes (Papanicolaou, 400×). Courtesy of J. Feng and S. Bandyopadhyay, Wayne State University, Detroit, MI. (**d**) A low-power view of the excision revealing a well-circumscribed and encapsulated lesion surrounded by unremarkable salivary gland tissue. The lesion consists of benign sebaceous glands intermixed and surrounded by benign lymphoid tissue mainly comprising small mature lymphocytes (hematoxylin and eosin, 10×). Courtesy of J. Feng and S. Bandyopadhyay, Wayne State University, Detroit, MI. (**e**) A higher power view of a tissue section exhibiting the benign sebaceous glands intermixed and surrounded by benign lymphoid tissue mainly comprising small mature lymphocytes (hematoxylin and eosin, 100×). Courtesy of J. Feng and S. Bandyopadhyay, Wayne State University, Detroit, MI.

lacks sebaceous glands, then it is termed lymphadenoma. The aspirate smears of sebaceous lymphadenoma contain islands of bland and benign sebaceous cells surrounded by benign-appearing predominantly small-sized lymphocytes (Figures 17.5b and c). The histological appearance is similar with obvious well circumscription (Figures 17.5d and e). To differentiate these tumors from metastatic carcinoma into intraparotid lymph node, sebaceous carcinoma, and lymphoepithelial carcinoma; the epithelial cells of lymphadenoma lack neoplastic features. Surgical excision is curative. In very rare occasions, sebaceous carcinoma can be observed or can develop in sebaceous lymphadenoma in which the epithelial sebaceous cells show malignant cytological features.

17.3.5   Ductal Papillomas

A group of benign papillomas develop from the major excretory ducts and encompasses the following entities: inverted ductal papilloma (IDP), intraductal papilloma (IP), and sialadenoma papilliferum (SAP). These tumors are rare and affect middle age and elderly patients and in general are characterized by the presence of bland cytological features and papillary architecture. They predominantly affect minor salivary glands with associated duct ectasia after partial or complete obstruction. IDP exhibits endophytic growth into duct lumina and occasionally forms nodular masses. The proliferating epithelium is squamous and sometimes basaloid squamous. Occasionally, goblet cells are present. Because of these cells, the major differential diagnosis is mucoepidermoid carcinoma, both on aspiration and tissue samples. Although IDPs are not encapsulated, they are well circumscribed and lack the infiltrative growth of mucoepidermoid carcinoma. Therefore, differentiating between these two diagnoses requires clinical, radiological, and histological examination. IP is a very rare, solitary benign intraductal papilloma causing solitary cyst dilatation that affects the minor salivary glands of the elderly. Histologically, the epithelium is columnar surrounding fibrovascular fronds. SAP is also a very rare benign tumor affecting mainly the hard and soft palate at middle age. Histologically, they are characterized by both exo- and endophytic components. The exophytic component consists of squamous proliferation with a papillary and verrucous architecture and an underlying more complex glandular proliferation. The glandular proliferation is variable with short cuboidal and tall columnar cells. Duct ectasia and interstitial fibrosis can also be present. FNA smears of these materials are rarely performed, but when they are done they will show predominantly benign bland papillae (Figure 17.6) in addition to other cellular components depending on the underlying diagnosis. Basically, a lack of infiltration and cellular and nuclear atypia in addition to absence of intermediate cells are clues to distinguish these from mucoepidermoid carcinoma.

17.3.6   Mucinous Adenocarcinoma

This tumor is rare and mainly affects the palate and sublingual glands and, from its name, predominantly consists of mucinous-producing and mucinous-containing tumor cells floating in abundant pools of mucin. The tumor cells can be single or in clusters occasionally surrounded by thin fibrous strands. Fine needle aspiration of such tumors should reveal mucin pools with cuboidal mildly atypical epithelial cells, some of which should be in clusters (Figure 17.7). Clear cytoplasm that contains mucin is expected. The differential diagnosis includes mucoepidermoid carcinoma and mucin-rich salivary duct carcinoma.

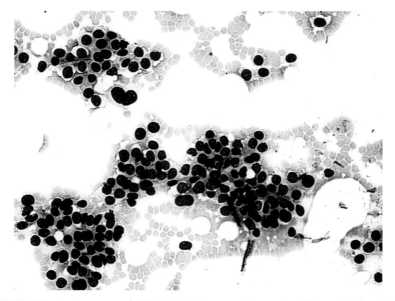

FIGURE 17.6. Aspirate smears of histologically proven inverted papilloma showing delicate papillae with bland cytological and nuclear features (MGG stain, 400×). Courtesy of J. Klijanienko, Institut Curie, Paris, France.

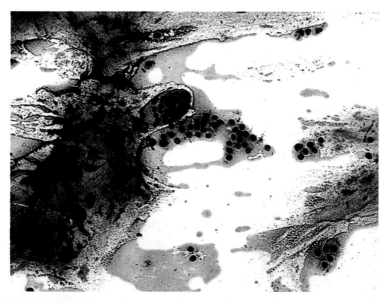

FIGURE 17.7. View of an aspirate smear from a primary mucinous adenocarcinoma of the parotid gland displaying single and clusters of mucin-containing tumor cells swimming in a pool of mucin characteristic of this tumor (MGG stain, 400×). Courtesy of J. Klijanienko, Institut Curie, Paris, France.

17.3.7 Adenocarcinoma, Not Otherwise Specified

By definition, this is probably a heterogeneous group of carcinomas that are primary salivary gland ductal adenocarcinomas morphologically different from any other well-characterized carcinomas of salivary glands. The diagnosis is mainly made on histological sections but can be suggested on cytological smears. Many believe that the frequency of such a diagnosis is diminishing because the criteria for other well-characterized adenocarcinomas are currently improving (Figure 17.8a–f).

17.3.8 Clear Cell Carcinoma, Not Otherwise Specified (Also Known as Hyalinzing Clear Cell Carcinoma)

Because many other salivary gland tumors can contain clear cells with varying degrees, this rare malignant epithelial tumor by definition should consist exclusively of clear cells. They mainly involve the intraoral minor salivary glands. The aspirate smears show a monotonous population of medium-size round-to-polygonal cells with clear cytoplasm arranged in

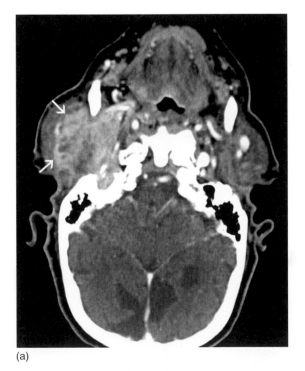

(a)

FIGURE 17.8. (*Continued*)

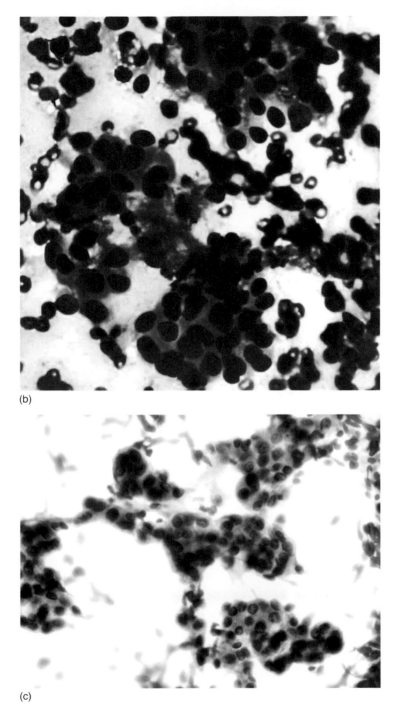

(b)

(c)

FIGURE 17.8. (*Continued*)

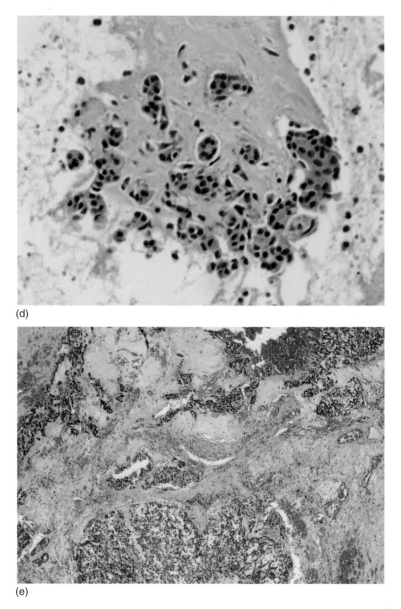

(d)

(e)

FIGURE 17.8. (*Continued*)

clusters and sometimes in sheets (Figure 17.9a). The nuclei are central or slightly eccentric with occasional small nucleoli. Histological examination recapitulates the smears with sheets and cords of cells with optically clear cytoplasm separated by fibrous strands (Figure 17.9b and c). The cytoplasm will stain with glycogen stains but not with mucin stain, an important feature

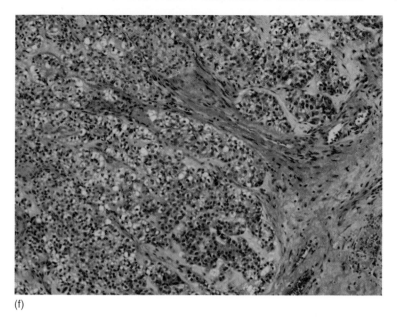

(f)

FIGURE 17.8. (**a**) A computed tomography scan image of a right parotid tumor for a patient who presented with an enhancing right parotid tumor and facial nerve paralysis. The tumor involves the whole gland and infiltrates the surrounding structures including skull base invasion with destruction. Courtesy of I. Zak, Wayne State University, Detroit, MI. (**b**) Aspirate smears at medium power revealing clusters of tumor cells with a mucoid and probably mucinous background. The cells are medium size, cuboidal, and slightly polygonal with slightly abundant cytoplasm and bland nuclei (Diff Quik, 400×). Courtesy of H. Saleh, Wayne State University, Detroit, MI. (**c**) The smears on a Papanicolaou stain showed clusters and papillary formation of medium size cells with occasional acini, bland nuclei, and small nucleoli (Papanicolaou, 400×). Courtesy of H. Saleh, Wayne State University, Detroit, MI. (**d**) The cell block section showed bland epithelial clusters of cells forming glands in either a thick mucinous background or a mucoid/myxoid matrix material background (hematoxylin and eosin, 200×). (**e**) A core biopsy showed a highly infiltrative epithelial tumor with necrosis, hemorrhage, and extensive perineural invasion shown here in the center of the photomicrograph (hematoxylin and eosin, 40×). (**f**) Another higher power section showing stromal infiltration with glandular tumor cells that have vacuolated cytoplasm (hematoxylin and eosin, 100×). Courtesy of H. Saleh, Wayne State University, Detroit, MI.

to differentiate this tumor from mucoepidermoid carcinoma and other carcinomas. Mitosis and ductal formations are absent. Prognosis is excellent after surgical removal. In addition to clinical and radiological data, immunohistochemical stains may be needed to rule out metastasis from clear cell renal cell carcinoma.

17.3.9 Small Cell Carcinoma

Also known as small undifferentiated carcinoma and neuroendocrine carcinoma, it is a very rare and aggressive primary tumor of salivary glands

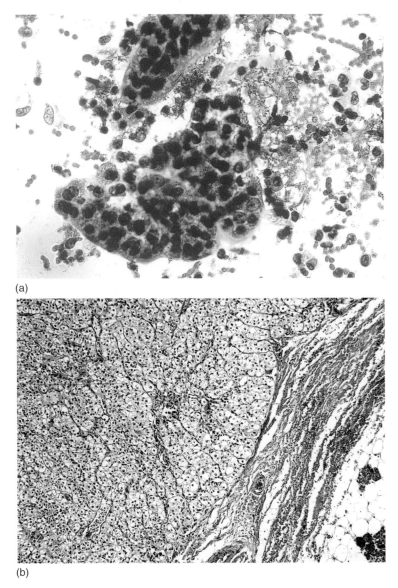

(a)

(b)

FIGURE 17.9. (*Continued*)

with morphology similar to lung small cell carcinoma. The tumor cells are small in size with scant cytoplasm and inconspicuous nucleoli (Figure 17.10). Clustering with molding and the characteristic "salt and pepper" chromatin are usually observed on the Papanicolaou stain. Although the immunoprofile is similar to their lung counterparts, they differ in that salivary gland small cell

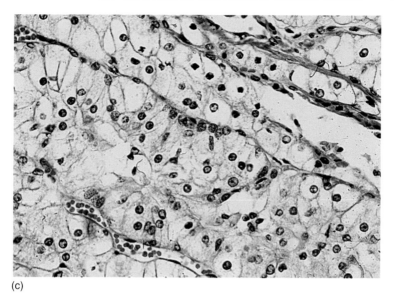

(c)

FIGURE 17.9. (**a**) A high-power view of an aspirate smear showing the clear cells in clusters. Nuclear atypia and occasional nucleoli are noted. (Papanicolaou stain, 600×). (**b**) On histological examination, the tumor consisted completely of cells with clear cytoplasm, small nuclei, and occasional small nucleoli. The features justified the diagnosis of clear cell carcinoma. No other malignancy was detected, and the tumor was considered primary (hematoxylin and eosin 100×). (**c**) A higher power examination showed that the tumor comprises completely of cords of clear cells and thin delicate septa in between (hematoxylin and eosin 400×). Courtesy of F. Abdul-Karim, University Hospitals Case Medical Center, Cleveland, OH.

carcinoma is commonly immunoreactive for cytokeratins 20, and they lack expression for thyroglobulin transcription factor-1 (TTF-1).

17.3.10 Carcinosarcoma

Carcinosarcoma is an extremely rare high-grade malignant tumor that contains both carcinoma and sarcoma components. They mainly affect major salivary glands with a predilection to the parotid. These tumors are highly infiltrative and harbor a poor prognosis. Some develop on top of preexisting pleomorphic adenoma. Their aspirate smears contain both carcinoma and sarcoma components.

17.3.11 Large Cell Carcinoma (Also Known as Large Cell Undifferentiated Carcinoma)

This carcinoma is a rare aggressive salivary gland tumor that affects mainly the major salivary glands and consists mainly of large pleomorphic tumor

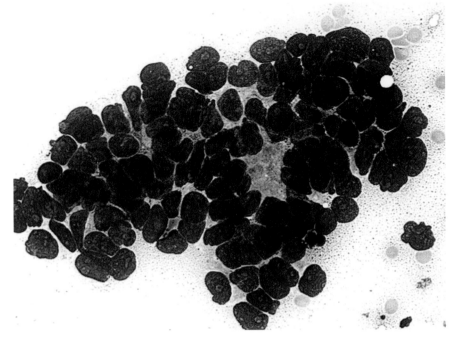

FIGURE 17.10. A high-power view of primary small cell carcinoma involving the parotid gland. The cytological features are similar to lung small cell carcinoma in which the tumor cells are small to medium in size with a high nuclear cytoplasmic ratio, indistinct nucleoli, and nuclear molding (MGG stain, 600×). Courtesy of J. Klijanienko, Institut Curie, Paris, France.

cells singly and in clusters. Fine needle aspirate smears exhibit large cells with abundant cytoplasm and pleomorphic nuclei with prominent nucleoli. Occasional multinucleated tumor giant cells are sometimes observed. The differential diagnosis includes lymphoma, melanoma, and other high-grade carcinomas. Immunoreactivity for cytokeratins and an absence of lymphoid and melanoma markers are usually needed to make the diagnosis. The absence of mucin on special stains helps to rule out mucoepidermoid carcinoma.

17.3.12   Lymphoepithelial Carcinoma (Also Known as Lymphoepithelioma-Like Carcinoma or Malignant Lymphoepithelial Lesion)

These tumors are rare and occur more commonly in certain geographic areas where they mainly involve major salivary glands. Like lymphoepithelial carcinoma in other organs, they consist of malignant epithelial cells embedded in lymphoid-rich stroma sometimes containing lymphoid follicles. The malignant epithelial cells are medium to large in size, observed forming islands or cords, and are immunoreactive for cytokeratins. The lymphoid cells are polyclonal in nature of both T and B lymphocytes and occasional plasma cells. A strong association with the Epstein-Barr virus is well known especially in endemic areas such as the Inuits (Eskimo) of the Arctic regions of Canada, Greenland, and Alaska.

Making the diagnosis solely on cytomorphology is difficult; using ancillary studies such as immunohistochemical stains and flow cytometry is critical.

17.3.13 Sialoblastoma

These tumors are very rare tumors of infancy and perinatal periods and affect the parotid and submandibular glands, and composed of primitive blastema cells. The cells are small to medium in size with very scant cytoplasm, hyperchromatic nuclei, and inconspicuous nucleoli. Two variable morphological variants embark on the behavior. The first is a basaloid bland blastoma that lacks significant atypia, necrosis, and increased mitosis; behaves in benign fashion; and can be cured by surgical removal. The second variant is malignant, aggressive blastoma with cellular atypia, necrosis, and frequent mitosis. A cytological description of this tumor is scarce in the literature. Basaloid cells in an infant with a salivary gland tumor are the clues.

17.3.14 Soft Tissue Tumors

Pure mesenchymal tumors of salivary glands are very rare. Benign tumors are more common than malignant, and the latter tend to occur in the elderly. Almost all soft tissue tumors have been reported in salivary glands. Among the benign neoplasms, the most frequent are hemangioma, lymphangioma, neurofibroma, schwannoma, lipoma, and fibrohistiocytic tumors. However, the sarcoma list includes, but is not limited to, haemangiopericytoma, malignant schwannoma, fibrosarcoma, and malignant fibrous histiocytoma.

ACKNOWLEDGMENT

I would like to thank all the colleagues who contributed images for this chapter, Drs. F. Abdul-Karim, N Aloudah, S. Bandyopadhyay, H. Cramer, J. Feng, J. Klijanienko, H. Saleh, and I. Zak.

RECOMMENDED READINGS

Apple SK, Moatamed NA, Lai CK, Bhuta S. Sebaceous adenoma of the parotid gland: a case report with fine needle aspiration findings and histologic correlation. Acta Cytol 2009;53:419–422.

Banich J, Reyes CV, Bier-Laning C. Sebaceous lymphadenoma identified by fine needle aspiration biopsy: a case report. Acta Cytol 2007;51:211–213.

Barnes L, Eveson JW, Reichart P, Sidransky D. Chapter 5. In: Pathology & Genetics, Head and Neck Tumours. WHO Classification of Tumours. Lyon, France: IARC Press; 2005. p 209–281.

Batsakis JG, el-Naggar AK, Luna MA. "Adenocarcinoma, not otherwise specified": a diminishing group of salivary gland carcinomas. Ann Otol Rhinol Laryngol 1992;10:102–104.

Bron LP, Traynor SJ, McNeil EB, O'Brien CJ. Primary and metastatic cancer of the parotid: comparison of clinical behavior in 232 cases. Laryngoscope 2003;113:1070–1075.

Buchner A, Merrell PW, Carpenter WM. Relative frequency of intra-oral minor salivary gland tumors: a study of 380 cases from northern California and comparison to reports from other parts of the world. L Oral Pathol Med 2007;36:207–214.

Castelino-Prabhu S, Li QK, Ali SZ. Nonsebaceous lymphadenoma of parotid gland: cytopathologic findings and differential diagnosis. Diagn Cytopathol 2010;38:137–140.

Cho KJ, Ro JY, Choi J, Choi SH, Nam SY, Kim Sy. Mesenchymal neoplasms of the major salivary glandsL clinicopathological features of 18 cases. Eur Arch Otorhinolaryngol 2008;265:S47–56.

Coitoru CM, Moonev JE, Luna MA. Sebaceous lymphadenocarcinoma of salivary glands. Ann Diagn Pathol 2003;7:236–239.

Eicher SA, Clayman GL, Myers JN, Gillenwater AM. A prospective study of intraoperative lymphatic mapping for head and neck cutaneous melanoma. Arch Otolaryngol Head Neck Surg 2002;128:241–246.

Elshenawy Y, Youngberg GA, Al-Abbadi MA. Unusual clinical presentation of cutaneous malignant melanoma metastatic to the parotid gland, initially discovered by fine needle aspiration. Case report and review of literature. Digan Cytopathol 2010. Forthcoming.

Dardick I, Thomas MJ. Lymphadenoma of parotid gland: two additional cases and a literature review. Oral Surg Oral Med Oral Pathol Oral Radiol Endod 2008;105:491–494.

Hruban RH, Erozan YS, Zinreich SJ, Kashima HK. Fine needle aspiration of monomorphic adenomas. Am J Clin Pathol 1988;90:46–51.

Javaram G, Peh SC. Lymphoepithelial carcinoma of salivary gland—cytologic, histologic, immunohistochemical, and in situ hybridization features in a case. Diagn Cytopathol 2000;22:400–402.

Karayianis SL, Francisco GJ, Schumann. Clinical utility of head and neck aspiration cytology. Diagn Cytopathol 1988;4:187–192.

Kim T, Yoon GS, Kim O, Gong G. Fine needle aspiration diagnosis of malignant mixed tumor (carcinosarcoma) arising in pleomorphic adenoma of salivary gland. A case report. Acta Cytol 1998;42:1027–1031.

Layfield LJ. Fine-needle aspiration in the diagnosis of head and neck lesions: a review and discussion of problems in differential diagnosis. Diagn Cytopathol. 2007;35:798–805.

Lussier C, Klijanienko J, Vielh P. Fine-needle aspiration of metastatic nonlymphomatous tumors to the major salivary glands: a clinicopathologic study of 40 cases cytologically diagnosed and histologically correlated. Cancer 2000;90:350–356.

Mair S, Phillips JI, Cohen R. Small cell undifferentiated carcinoma of the parotid gland. Cytologic, histologic, immunohistochemical and ultrastructural features of a Neuroendocrine variant. Acta Cytol 1989;33:164–168.

Malata CM, Camilleri IG, McLean NR, Piggot TA, Kelly CG, Chippindalet AJ, Soamesf JV. Malignant tumours of the parotid gland: a 12-year review. Br J Plast Surg 1997;50:600–608.

Moore JG, Bocklage T. Fine-needle aspiration biopsy of large-cell undifferentiated carcinoma of the salivary glands: presentation of two cases, literature review, and differential cytodiagnosis of high-grade salivary gland malignancies. Diagn Cytopathol 1998;19:44–50.

Prayson RA, Sebek BA. Parotid gland malignant melanomas. Arch Pathol Lab Med. 2000;124:1780–1784.

Wang B, Brandwein M, Gordon R, Robinson R, Urken M, Zarbo RJ. Primary salivary clear cell tumors—a diagnostic approach: a clinicopathologic and immunohistochemical study of 20 patients with clear cell carcinoma, clear cell myoepithelial carcinoma, and epithelial-myoepithelial carcinoma. Arch Pathol Lab Med 2002;126:676–685.

Williams SB, Ellis GL, Warnock GR. Sialoblastoma: a clinicopathologic and immunohistochemical study of 7 cases. Ann Diagn Pathol 2006;10:320–326.

Yang S, Zhang J, Chen X, Wang L, Xie F. Clear cell carcinoma, not otherwise specified, of salivary glands: a clinicopathologic study of 4 cases and review of the literature. Oral Surg Oral Med Oral Pathol Oral Radiol Endod 2008;106:712–720.

INDEX

Salivary Gland Cytology: A Color Atlas, Edited by Mousa A. Al-Abbadi
Copyright © 2011 Wiley-Blackwell